SKIN HEALTHY

Everyone's Guide to
Great Skin

Norman Levine, M.D.

TAYLOR PUBLISHING COMPANY
Dallas, Texas

*To my wife, Carol, who has done the impossible;
she has raised our two children while keeping
her sanity, grace, and sense of humor.*

*To Bonnie and Brian, who have always
made it interesting around our home.*

Copyright © 1995 by Norman Levine

Published by Taylor Publishing Company
         1550 West Mockingbird Lane
         Dallas, Texas 75235

Library of Congress Cataloging-in-Publication Data

Levine, Norman, 1945 Mar. 18–
      Skin healthy : everyone's guide to great skin / Norman Levine.
          p.   cm.
      Includes index.
      ISBN 0-87833-900-0 (pbk.)
      1. Skin—Care and hygiene.   I. Title.
RL87.L43   1995
616.5—dc20   95-9070
                                                                 CIP

Printed in the United States of America

10   9   8   7   6   5   4   3   2   1

Contents

Introduction

T he health care world is evolving rapidly. One of the major changes is less on-demand specialty care available because it is viewed (incorrectly) by many third-party payers as not being cost effective. This leads many to seek care from primary care physicians, who know something about all medical specialties but are not experts in any one discipline. The only alternative may be to fend for oneself. The elements of routine skin care and the management of many common skin problems do not require an advanced degree. In fact, with a little direction many skin conditions can be resolved without ever seeing a specialist or any other physician. This book will provide you with the information to handle many of these problems by yourself. It will also explode a number of popular myths about the skin and how it functions.

I am a practicing dermatologist as well as an academician. I strongly believe that the practitioners of my specialty can be of great service to you. I will detail many circumstances in which a trip to the dermatologist can improve the quality of your skin, and often the quality of your life as well. Not all skin diseases require the services of a specialist, however. After reading this book, you will be able to determine for yourself whether it is worth your while to consult a dermatologist or whether watchful waiting and inexpensive over-the-counter medications will solve your problem.

A recurrent theme in this book is that it is *your* body; you should be able to make informed choices about what is in your best interest. A physician can outline therapeutic alternatives that might be of benefit to you, but it is your right and responsibility to decide what is appropriate for your particular situation. The days of lying passively on the exam table and awaiting the doctor's dictum from on high are rapidly drawing to a close. The knowledge that you gain from this book will enable you to become an active participant in your health care.

The tone of this book may be different from what you might expect from a physician. The irreverence, humor, skepticism, and even a little sarcasm are not accidental. They reflect my overall approach to life as well as to the practice of medicine. In addition, I want you to understand that skin care is not a mysterious undertaking in which all knowledge is held by a privileged few. The concepts put forward in this book are not difficult to grasp, and with information comes power. As an informed individual, you will be empowered to make important choices about your personal health care.

1

Dermatology and You

It's Monday morning and you bounce out of bed ready for another tough week of work. You scramble into the bathroom and check yourself out in the mirror. To your horror, a giant zit the size of a golf ball has landed on your nose and threatens to take over. It's tempting to pop it and hope the house doesn't need to be fumigated afterward. But wait, didn't you read somewhere that the self-manipulation of pimples could lead to meningitis and death?

There is no way you can be seen in public with this new appendage on your nose. You have to see a doctor, but who is the right person for this delicate job? Contrary to what you might think, the answer to that question is not simple. In choosing a care giver (the new, politically correct term for anyone who makes a living by treating other people's infirmities), there are a number of factors that need to be considered. In this chapter, you will learn how to find the right doctor for your skin problem and survive the maze of an office visit. You will learn to come armed with a few very valuable bits of information, expect to be a bit manhandled, ask questions, follow instructions, and respect but not worship your doctor.

If you open the telephone book in any medium or large city, there will be many physicians to choose from. Virtually any doctor is allowed to treat skin disease, but there may be a tremendous difference in knowledge between individuals, depending on training, experience, and interest. The majority of medical schools teach dermatology to their students, but this training is usually rudimentary and not helpful in the real world, especially if a doctor doesn't keep up to date.

Fledgling physicians learn the bulk of what they will use in practice during the course of a residency. Depending on the specialty, the doctor spends two to seven years in a training program learning the craft. Certain specialty programs train their residents to be primary care physicians; these people are the family doctors who treat all types of uncomplicated ailments. Most of these programs teach at least something about the care of skin disease. Internists are specially trained physicians who mainly concern themselves with nonsurgical disorders of the internal organs. Many internists function as primary care doctors, and some training programs include at least some exposure to skin problems. Pediatricians limit their practices to the care of children. Since there are many pediatric skin problems, most of these physicians learn how to treat minor skin conditions in children. Other specialists usually avoid skin disease at all costs because they do not feel comfortable dealing with weird rashes. When pressed, these people know four or five skin diseases and two or three treatments, which they use for all skin problems.

Should you trust your skin to your family physician? It depends on the nature of your problem and the level of interest and expertise of the physician. You might call the office first and ask the nurse or receptionist if the doctor likes to treat skin conditions. If the answer is yes and it is a minor ailment, you might try him before going to a specialist.

Many people trust their health care to nontraditional health professionals such as naturopaths, reflexologists, chiropractors, and nutritionists. As a physician who cares for skin disease all the time, my semi-unbiased opinion is that these people know little about the nature of cutaneous disease (a disease affecting the skin) and that most of the medications they prescribe are placebos. (If you believe that wearing your college beanie helps push your alma mater's football team to victory, you understand what a placebo response is.)

If your doctor gets slightly nauseated at the thought of treating unsightly skin eruptions, you might consider going to a dermatologist. Anyone who finishes medical school and does one postgraduate year of internship can be licensed to practice medicine and call himself whatever he wants, including "El Supremo Dermatologist." This does not mean that he knows any more than your family practitioner. One way to ensure that you are treated by a physician with special training in diseases of the skin is to select one who has completed an approved residency. It is best if he has passed a qualifying examination, making him a board-certified specialist. You can find out the credentials of a practitioner by calling the office and asking the receptionist. If she doesn't know or won't tell you, excuse yourself and hang up quickly. The local medical society may also have this information, but it should not be necessary to call there often.

Once you've determined that your prospective dermatologist is board certified, if you are really inquisitive, you might ask what training program he graduated from. In most instances, if you have heard of the institution, that is probably good enough. Many small, lesser-known programs produce outstanding dermatologists, but there is not any way that you are going to be able to determine this without some serious background investigation.

The vast majority of physicians who complete dermatology training know what they are doing. Still, there are differences in character, judgment, knowledge, manual dexterity, bedside manner, fee schedules, and availability. To fine tune your choice, you might solicit the advice of your family doctor who may know how a given person practices. This is not foolproof, however, since personal friendships, business relationships, old gambling debts, and other factors may color his opinion. If you asked me to pick an ophthalmologist for you, it is likely that I would give you the name of my friend. He is a very nice fellow and he usually lets me beat him in tennis, but I don't really know his level of competence in his specialty.

For 95% of all skin conditions, almost any well-trained dermatologist will be able to handle the situation easily. So it often becomes a matter of personal preference. Sometimes the best person to ask about a doctor is a trusted friend or family member who has already seen him. These people may not be experts in evaluating clinical competence, but most reasonably astute observers can distinguish a caring and compassionate person from one who has other motivations for practicing medicine. I often marvel at the fact that certain doctors whose abilities are not of the highest caliber have large practices full of satisfied patients. Could it be that these practitioners are actually kind to their patients and please them in ways that are not measured with tests of knowledge?

What kinds of problems should you bring to the dermatologist, and how is he equipped to handle them? A specialist in skin diseases deals with conditions of the skin surface, the mucous membranes (the lining of the mouth, genitals, and anus), the hair, and the nails. Most dermatologists can be considered general practitioners of the skin, but there are people with special areas of expertise within dermatology. Many dermatologists, for example, have acquired exceptional surgical skills. They can perform complex procedures, including skin grafts and flaps, facial peels, hair transplantation, and aggressive skin cancer

surgery. In chapter 8, I discuss more about the specifics of these procedures. Suffice it to say that if you have a growth that needs to be
removed, most dermatologists can perform that procedure for you.

Why have a dermatologist do these things when the world is populated with skilled plastic surgeons? Plastic surgeons and surgically
inclined dermatologists do many of the same procedures. Plastic surgeons will often handle "bigger" cases in which general anesthesia is
required or structures other than the skin are involved, such as nasal
reconstructions (nose jobs) and breast augmentations. To become pro-
ficient in these techniques, plastic surgeons must undergo a long and
arduous training program, much more rigorous than what dermatologists are subjected to. The ultimate results might be identical whether
a good dermatologist or a good plastic surgeon does the work. The
major advantage that the dermatologic surgeon has over the plastic
surgeon is that he is more familiar with skin diseases and may have a
better understanding of the treatment options.

If money is no object or you are a famous movie star, go to a plastic surgeon for any little growth that you want removed. If you are like
the rest of us, consider a competent dermatologist with a special interest in skin surgery for your routine procedures. A few dermatologists
spend an extra year or two in special surgery fellowships. Most of
these individuals acquire exceptional dermatologic surgical skills. It
may cost more to have one of these people operate on you, but in complicated cases, it is well worth it.

If one of your children develops a skin condition and a pediatri-
cian can't handle the particular problem, most general dermatologists
feel quite comfortable in dealing with these situations. There are a few
dermatologists with extra training and experience in pediatric dermatology; some of these individuals have been trained in both pediatrics
and dermatology. In more complicated cases it might be worthwhile to
get on an airplane and fly to wherever these people practice, which is
usually in an academic center. A severe case of pimples in an anxious
teenager does not qualify for a cross-country flight.

There are times when the diagnosis of a skin problem is not obvious; in these situations, laboratory tests are needed. One common way
that additional information is obtained is by examining skin tissue
taken from the affected area. This is called a skin biopsy. All dermatologists are trained to examine skin biopsies under the microscope and
make diagnoses based on what is seen. Many will continue to do this in
their practices if they feel competent to do so. However, for tough
cases, there are referral centers where pathologists perform this service. Some pathologists have obtained extra training in the examina-

tion of skin specimens and may have both dermatology and additional dermatopathology training. If a skin biopsy is ever performed on you and your doctor is sending the specimen elsewhere, insist that a specially trained dermatopathologist examine the specimen. General pathologists know a great deal but many do not have much experience in skin pathology.

If I had my choice of a person to interpret a tough case under a microscope, I would want someone who is both a dermatologist and a dermatopathologist. How do you find out who your doctor sends his skin biopsy specimens to? Ask him. I guarantee that he will be surprised at the question, and you may even convince him to send your specimen to an expert if he doesn't already.

After considering your options, you have decided that the thing on your nose needs the attention of a dermatologist. You make an appointment and begin the countdown to when the doctor will miraculously make the pimple disintegrate. This is a nice story, but will it really happen? Will you be greeted by warm smiles and a cozy, comfortable waiting room, or a drafty place with uncomfortable chairs and nasty receptionists and nurses? Should you be prepared to write your memoirs while waiting to see the doctor or be ready to be whisked into the examination room for immediate attention? Frankly, I have no idea what will happen to you since physicians practice in many different ways. However, I will give you some notion of what to expect from a typical visit to a dermatologist's office.

When you enter the office, go to the reception desk before sitting down. That way the staff will know that you have arrived. Patients have been known to take root in waiting rooms because no one was aware of their presence. You will most likely be asked for some insurance information. It is a good idea to have available the wallet-sized cards that insurers issue. Even if you think that this particular office visit is not covered by your insurance plan, give the receptionist the information anyway. The insurance rules are complex and variable. Certain services that the doctor performs for you might qualify for reimbursement even if the charge for the office visit itself is not covered.

Many physicians ask all new patients to fill out a medical history form. This form outlines your medical history, including drug allergies, major illnesses, current medications, and, finally, the chief complaint that brings you to see the doctor. It is extremely important that this history is as complete as possible, even if it takes a few extra minutes. Picture this horror story: A patient forgets to note on the questionnaire that she is allergic to penicillin. The doctor prescribes this antibiotic under a different name so the patient is not aware that she is getting a drug that might cause an adverse reaction. She takes the medication and proceeds to give new meaning to the phrase, "She's as red as a lobster, and she feels like one too."

Dermatologists often schedule up to eight or ten patients an hour, and even give two or three different people the same appointment time. Don't frustrate yourself by comparing appointment times with other patients in the waiting room. It will only annoy you and probably will not get you seen any faster. Depending on the physician, expect at least a ten-minute wait. If you hate cooling your heels, try getting the first appointment of the day; then you are more likely to be seen with only a minimal delay. You might also call about thirty minutes before the time of your appointment and ask if the doctor is running on schedule. If he is an hour late, ask the receptionist if you may arrive a little later. Be careful about using this little maneuver because some offices secretly use a "first come, first served" approach, regardless of what the schedule says.

Once you are escorted into the exam room, you may be asked to disrobe. I know that you only have a zit on your nose, but on first visits many dermatologists prefer to do a complete examination of the skin to establish a baseline condition against which any future changes can be compared. Many potentially serious skin problems have been uncovered by this simple procedure. If your doctor doesn't ask to examine your entire skin surface, consider suggesting it to him; he'll be happy to accommodate your wishes.

If you are modest you can refuse the offer for a complete examination, but this would be a big mistake on your part. If you are uncomfortable with the complete skin exam, request a "sun-exposed" skin exam. This includes all areas of the skin except where it would be difficult to tan without being a dedicated nudist. This type of exam is particularly helpful in detecting common skin cancers that usually appear in sites that have had a great deal of sun exposure (more about that later). If you happen to be a woman and your new dermatologist is a man, expect to have his nurse in the room as a chaperone. If there is not a nurse in the room, you are well within your rights to ask for one.

There is no set "uniform" you should expect your new doctor to be wearing. Depending on the customs of the area and the individual's personal style, he may be wearing a suit or a sport coat (too formal for my part of the country but quite common in the Midwest), a white coat, or everyday dress. If your tastes go to the really informal, you can probably find a dermatologist somewhere who wears shorts and a T-shirt with a picture of the Grateful Dead on it. Some people have a certain image of a doctor. If this is one of your hangups, call ahead and ask the receptionist what to expect. As times have changed, doctors today tend to dress more like you and less like your grandfather.

For routine problems, the length of the first office visit is rarely over fifteen minutes, unless a procedure is being performed, such as a skin biopsy or surgical removal of a growth. During that short appointment, the physician will ask for a *succinct* history of your ailment. A dermatology office visit is different from one to your family doctor. It is much more focused on the skin problem; often, your other medical conditions are given short shrift. This is not because the doctor isn't interested; rather, experienced practitioners learn to exclude irrelevant information so that the nature of the chief problem is not clouded. As much as the dermatologist would like to chat with you about the trick knee that you got while you were playing Pee Wee football in 1954, if it isn't germane to the present illness, he may try to move the discussion to more relevant topics.

Once the physician has made the diagnosis, he will sit down with you and discuss the problem and will probably prescribe a medication. Occasionally, he will give you samples of the drug he wishes you to use. For minor problems, the condition might clear with the use of the samples without your ever having to fill the prescription. In most situations, you will need more medication than is in the small sample tubes. Don't fill the prescription until you have tried the samples, in case you develop an adverse reaction to the medication. Don't hesitate to ask your doctor for starter packages if he does not offer them.

Many dermatologists will provide printed material to supplement what they tell you. Since it is impossible to remember all the things that the doctor said to you, these fact-filled information sheets are often invaluable to refresh your memory about aspects of your skin problem and its therapy. Again, you ought to ask for these materials; your doctor will be happy to supply them to you if they are available for your particular condition.

There are times when all that you hope could be accomplished in a single office visit simply can't be done. This is particularly true if a surgical procedure needs to be performed. Often, the details of the operation will be discussed, and it will be scheduled for the near future. This allows the physician to block out sufficient time to handle your needs without being pressured by a waiting room full of irate patients. In addition, you may have to get pre-operative laboratory tests or arrange for transportation after the procedure.

Once the visit is completed, you will be given what is often called a superbill. It lists your diagnosis and itemizes the cost of the care that was delivered. You may not think the charges are so "super," but you should take this to the front desk and give it to the receptionist. Be prepared to pay at this time. The days of doctors not wanting to discuss financial matters in the office are long since gone. Don't expect to be billed later. This is a costly and inefficient way of doing business. If for some reason you are unable to pay at the time of service, be sure to discuss this with the front office staff or with the doctor *before* your appointment. Many offices will arrange a payment schedule that can fit within your budget. If it suits your needs, you might want to find out if they take credit cards for payment; many physicians do.

If you are a participant in an insurance plan that covers some or all of the cost of your care, some physicians will bill the plan for you and not require you to pay up front. However, most believe that it is a matter between you and the insurance carrier and it is your responsibility to collect from it. It is still the doctor's obligation to complete whatever forms are necessary so that you will be reimbursed.

Many people are enrolling in prepaid medical plans where monthly premiums substitute for a fee-for-service arrangement. In many programs, you will be required to receive prior authorization before you can see a specialist in consultation. That is something that you must arrange with your primary care provider *before* you make the dermatology appointment. Don't expect these plans to authorize payment for these services retroactively. They almost never do this. Your dermatologist is not being a hardhearted person by insisting that you pay your bill rather than waiting and hoping that he will be paid by your health plan, which has absolutely no contractual obligation to cover these charges.

Many plans have a co-pay provision that requires the patient to make a small payment at each visit. This is done to discourage frivolous trips to the doctor and to save the plan a little money. Don't try to weasel out of the five-dollar charge by feigning ignorance of this provision in your contract with the insurance company.

For those who have Medicare coverage, there are rapidly evolving and extremely complex rules about what services are covered and what the reimbursement will be for these services. One thing is clear: if your doctor is a participant in the Medicare program, he must accept the fee schedule for that program and not charge you more than what Medicare will pay. However, the program only pays 80% of the total, and the law clearly states that you must be charged the remaining 20% of the bill. Unless there is a profound reason you cannot pay this part of your tab, don't ask your doctor to become a lawbreaker by foregoing the collection of this amount.

A visit to a dermatologist can be pleasant and productive. The whole process can move so fast that, before you know it, you are in the car on the way home with a vague feeling that you don't know much more about your skin disease than before you arrived. The following are some tips to maximize your office visit.

Get your story straight. Give some thought to the chronology of events that may be directly associated with your present skin problem. If necessary, outline it in writing and give this to the doctor to read even before he begins questioning you. There is little that is more disconcerting than to have a patient whose story throws the doctor off the track because of inconsistencies or inaccuracies. I teach medical students, and as a part of their training they are asked to question the patient first and then come out of the room and report the story to me. I always find it humorous when I go into the room with the student and in her presence (and to her chagrin) the patient tells an entirely different tale to me. Please give the doctor or doctor-in-training a break and try to organize the history of the problem beforehand.

If you have seen other practitioners for your skin problem, try to obtain copies of these records. This is helpful for several reasons. Your present dermatologist can trace the course of your illness and find out what treatment has been used in the past. In addition, if skin biopsies or laboratory tests have been performed, your doctor may avoid having to repeat these tests. Last, if you really want to spice up your doctor's day and make a good impression on him, show him the old billing slips from the other physician. Many doctors have an almost morbid curiosity about what their colleagues charge for their services.

If you have several skin problems, write them down so that all of them can be addressed. An exam room sometimes seems intimidating, and many people get flustered to the point that they forget exactly why they made the appointment in the first place. Don't let the audible groan that you hear from the harried physician when he sees your list deter you from going through all the points before you leave. You are paying good money for the time and you deserve to have all of your concerns addressed. I can assure you of one thing—once you leave that examination room and the doctor has moved on to the next patient, getting his full attention again will be almost impossible. If you suddenly remember that you didn't show him something that worries you and rush in from the parking lot to discuss it, he may pretend that he doesn't even recognize you.

Be prepared to make some quick decisions. Most modern physicians have learned to respect the intelligence of their patients and often bring them right into the center of the decision-making process. In many instances, there is no single treatment of choice. Depending on the circumstances, one of several alternatives might be reasonable. Thus, you might be asked to be the ultimate decision maker. If after listening to the treatment possibilities you cannot decide, tell the doctor and he will probably ask you to call him when you have made a decision. This is perfectly reasonable and you should not have to apologize to anybody because you are not yet sure what is best for you.

If you do not feel competent to decide or if you wish to transfer the responsibility to the doctor, tell him so. Please remember that in many instances, only you know what's best for your particular situation. There will be instances where there is only one good option. Here, your doctor will do what he thinks is appropriate after explaining to you all the consequences of the treatment.

If you do not understand the explanation that your doctor provides, don't hide your ignorance because you think it might reflect badly on you. Speak up and ask that he talk in ordinary English. You are not a physician and there is no reason you should be expected to be an expert in dermatology any more than I can be expected to know what a computer whiz is talking about when he tries to explain RAM memory and SLIP-emulators.

If you return home and have additional questions, or if you have new concerns about the treatment program, call the doctor. Physicians expect to hear from some patients; that is part of the job. Sometimes it might be useful if a family member is also on the telephone line so that the two of you can compare notes afterward.

Be prepared to negotiate. Sometimes the dermatologist is on a completely different wavelength regarding what you want. Doctors get good at reading body language in a hurry, and this is often the only means that they have to assess a patient's desires. I might think that a little dot on your face has no medical or aesthetic consequence, while your perception is that the tumor is so huge that you can barely see around it. Without your input I would probably pass on it altogether. You need to convey clearly that you *want the bump gone now*. Don't wait for an invitation to express your views.

If your doctor is still reluctant to remove the lesion, (a lesion is a general term for any abnormality on the skin), explain why you believe that treatment is necessary. In turn, your doctor will probably give his reasons why therapy might not be in your best interest. This simple give-and-take usually leads to a satisfactory conclusion. There may be instances where your physician recommends that he do something that you would rather not have done. Again, you should discuss the pros and cons with him and reach some kind of accommodation. Always remember, it is *your* body and you have the final say in what ultimately happens. Never get railroaded into a course of action against your wishes because of your fear of upsetting the doctor or appearing stubborn. On the other hand, you must trust his judgment to some extent and rely on his experience and wisdom. He really does know more about your skin than your mother-in-law, Ann Landers, Oprah, or other individuals who might advise you about matters that are not necessarily in their realm of expertise.

There are circumstances when you and your doctor cannot agree on a plan for your care. Then it is time for a second opinion from another practitioner. Most physicians welcome this approach as a way of (1) allowing you a chance to explore all options, (2) showing you that they were right after all, or (3) getting contentious patients out of the office.

Be prepared to admit that the office visit was a disaster. In the vast majority of cases, patients are satisfied with the care that they receive from their dermatologist. There are rare instances where, for whatever reason, there are such bad vibrations between doctor and patient that dueling pistols might be the only way to resolve the situation. If it happens, try to realize it quickly and call a halt to the ordeal by making a quick exit.

Some patients feel guilty that they are "abandoning" the doctor. There is absolutely no rational reason for feeling this way. Your children, not your doctors, are on this earth to give you pangs of guilt. I have had patients refuse to allow me to contact their former dermatologist to obtain old records for fear of offending him. This attitude is totally unwarranted. I have some news for you: Patients are moving from physician to physician all the time and doctors do not even give it a second thought.

Most encounters that a patient has with a physician are perfectly straightforward, with an honest and conscientious care giver trying to do his best to improve the lot of the patient. There are a few circumstances where it does not work out that way. In the next few paragraphs I will introduce you to a few potentially dicey situations where you might want to watch your wallet. I am not saying that all who indulge in these practices are crooked; just be careful because they present the possibility for a conflict of interest.

Office laboratories. This is an unusual occurrence in dermatology offices. Since so few laboratory tests are ordered, it would be difficult to justify doing routine testing on enough patients to make it a worthwhile endeavor. If you should happen to need laboratory tests performed, ask your doctor to recommend two or three laboratories so that there will be no possible taint of impropriety.

Office dispensaries of medications. This practice really makes me nervous. I think that it would be almost impossible for a doctor to avoid the temptation to prescribe what he has for sale. For the convenience of the patient, the one-stop-shop approach to medical care is introduced. Presumably, the costs are competitive with your neighborhood drugstore, so what is the problem? Your biggest concern should be whether the doctor is doing a little end-of-the-month drug clearance with you as the clearancee. Perhaps you need all eight of the different medicines that he prescribes for your facial wrinkles, but if he sends you elsewhere to purchase them, you can rest a bit better knowing that he is not profiting directly from the transaction.

There are special circumstances where direct drug dispensing is not only useful but may be necessary. Some unusual or complex formulations are not available in pharmacies. In these situations, the dermatologist must contract with an outside laboratory or pharmaceutical wholesaler to prepare these drugs. Out of necessity, he must sell them to you in his office. Be advised that almost all medications can be bought from your local pharmacy. Regional wholesalers can supply the medication within two or three days if your medication is not in stock.

Frequent revisit theory. For many routine skin problems, one or two visits can set you on the right path toward a resolution of the problem. There are some situations, such as severe or chronic diseases or cases in which a potentially risky therapy is being used, when frequent monitoring is important for good medical care. However, weekly checkups for acne or routine follow-ups for problems that are already solved are examples of worrisome overutilization of the medical system. Consider discussing the situation with your doctor if you are such a frequent visitor to his office that you can spot new growth on the waiting room plants or your name is embossed in gold on one of the waiting room chairs.

Miracle doctors. Don't trust doctor number nine if he claims to have the magic answer and tells you that dermatologists numbers one through eight weren't smart enough to figure it out. There are very few secrets in modern medicine, and since most dermatologists are well trained and well read there is a large pool of general knowledge. If eight physicians haven't figured out your problem, you have probably reached the point of diminishing returns by seeking out number nine. There are many exceptions to this rule, but be careful, especially if you move on to nonconventional therapists who may make claims and promises that will be difficult to keep.

The notion that care givers can't make you better is sometimes a difficult and painful one to accept. There are times when letting nature decide the fate of a skin problem is the best route to follow. In future chapters, when I discuss the diagnosis and treatment of many common ailments, you will be surprised (and maybe a bit appalled) at the number of conditions for which there is no completely effective remedy.

Your doctor assumes many responsibilities when he accepts you as a patient. He must be compassionate, polite, attentive, solicitous of your needs and desires, and scrupulously honest. You also have certain responsibilities that should be discharged if you are to fulfill your end of the unwritten bargain that has been struck with your new doctor. A visit to the physician is different from a trip to Saks Fifth Avenue, where the customer is always right and can behave any way that he wishes without any consequence. Here is an unofficial code of conduct for you to consider:

- Try to be on time for your appointments. I know that your doctor might be chronically behind in his schedule, but you can help to minimize the problem for your fellow patients rather than compound it by being tardy yourself. If you see that there is no way that you are going to get to the office at the appointed time, call ahead and inform the receptionist. She will really appreciate that small courtesy.

- Don't be a no-show. The physician's office is not like an airline or a restaurant where they factor in all the people who they assume will not keep their reservations when assembling the day's roll. If your rash gets better or if you have decided to try that do-it-yourself kit, please call and cancel your appointment (more than ten minutes in advance). Many busy practices have waiting lists of patients who would die (not literally) to see the dermatologist a little sooner if there were an unexpected opening. Allow them this opportunity to get their care by canceling in advance.

- Don't complain about your former doctors. Nothing is less productive or more boring to one doctor than to hear that one of his esteemed colleagues is a clod. In the best of worlds, it is useless information. In the worst of worlds, your new doctor will assume that you are fully capable of saying the same things about him if all does not go smoothly. This might tend to make the doctor a tad defensive, and you definitely don't want a defensive doctor.

- If it is humanly possible, leave your screaming child in the waiting room (or better yet, at home). You should be the center of attention as a patient. If your child is crying, nagging, or taking flying leaps off the exam table, it detracts from the quality of the encounter. The best strategy is to bring along a mother's helper or an older sibling to occupy the little tyke in the waiting room. If this cannot be arranged, carry diversions that can occupy your child while you are evaluated. As a rule, never leave a small child unattended in the doctor's waiting room. Bad things can happen.

- Don't expect miracles or ask for them. There are times when the doctor cannot supply you with all the answers to your questions or is unable make everything all right. This can be frustrating, but try to avoid taking it out on the poor doctor. One of the least appreciated comments that an annoyed patient can make to a physician is, "Gee, if they can send a man to the moon why can't they figure out a way to..." Contrary to public opinion, rocket science is simple; clearing big zits on the face of a teenager in five or six minutes is quite difficult. If you would like to remedy the man-to-the-moon versus zit-cure dichotomy, write to your congressman and insist that money earmarked for NASA be diverted to the National Institutes of Health for dermatologic research. You are called a "patient" for a good reason. There are times when your doctor will call on you to be very patient, indeed. Skin diseases often clear slowly. This is frustrating to all concerned but is a fact of life. Try to be philosophical and accept what is not known as a challenge for the future. We should all take a cue from the elderly patient from the Bronx who, when informed that she had an incurable but relatively benign skin disease, exclaimed, "Thank God it isn't cancer."

  Before 1920, the role of the physician was to diagnose an illness and give the patient some idea of the prognosis. Physicians were widely respected for their skills in this regard, and patients were satisfied with this service. Since there were precious few effective remedies, doctors were not expected to cure much of anything. In the succeeding decades there have been major advances in medical technology; now, many conditions can be improved or cured with myriad therapies. Along with these advances have come increased expectations, some well justified and some entirely unrealistic. Dermatology is still at the stage where *no* treatment is the best course of action for hundreds of skin conditions. Be prepared to get this verdict from your dermatologist. It is not his fault, or anybody's fault for that matter, that this is the present situation in medicine. I have had patients threaten to refuse to pay their bill because "the doctor didn't do anything for me." In many situations, no therapy is better than some crackpot nostrum which costs good money and doesn't have any therapeutic benefit.

- Follow instructions. If you have made the commitment to place your trust in a physician, give yourself the full benefit of his care by doing what he suggests. There are good reasons why certain medications are used twice daily, not once a day and not three times a day. If a little treatment works well, it does not mean that much more of the same treatment will work that much better. If the instructions are to put a thin film of cream on a rash, all the extra material that you slather on never gets absorbed into the skin and is essentially useless. If a treatment course is ten days and you think that five or six days is enough, your eruption may clear temporarily only to rear its ugly head somewhere down the road.

  Under the general rubric of following instructions, never share your medications with others. Not all creams are alike and not all skin eruptions respond to the same medications. Here is a brief cautionary tale: An effective acne remedy is given to a boy whose acne does extremely well. He is so pleased that he shares the drug with his girlfriend, who happens to be pregnant at the time. The drug is well known to cause serious fetal abnormalities, and their baby is born with multiple major birth defects.

- Your last responsibility to your doctor is to avoid the temptation to steal the waiting room magazines. Many doctors seem rich and able to afford to buy more reading material for the waiting room, but it is incredibly annoying to walk out at the end of the day and find that the only magazines left on the rack are 1976 issues of *Soldier of Fortune* and *Modern Maturity*. If you are in the middle of an important article about Burt and Loni in *People* magazine and are unceremoniously interrupted by the nurse and asked to come to the exam room, ask the receptionist to photocopy the article for you. Most offices would be happy to do this to keep their magazine collection intact.

2

An Overview of the Skin

The skin appears to be only a covering for the body, with little function other than to keep what is inside from leaking out. Actually, the skin is the largest and one of the most complicated organs in the body. It has evolved to perform many important tasks that are absolutely critical to survival. Its structure is beautifully suited to withstand most environmental insults and to maintain internal equilibrium.

About now, you may be starting to nod off or are thinking of checking the table of contents for subjects that seem more interesting and important to your health. Why read about the beauties of a part of your anatomy that seems pretty boring? Who cares about how the skin is put together and how it functions? Before you leaf past this chapter, let me tell you why it is important to introduce some of the scientific principles surrounding the skin to you.

All of us are bombarded with claims from drug and cosmetic marketers that are supposedly supported with scientific data. Many of these turn out to be ridiculous once one applies some simple knowledge about the workings of the skin. In chapter 3, I will discuss cellulite, a truly bogus concept that has made its way into the health lexicon. Cellulite is supposed to be some evil curse on middle-aged women with extra money to spare on questionable products. Presumably, it consists of abnormal fat deposits under the skin. Cosmetic manufacturers would like you to believe that these deposits can be reduced by applying special products that penetrate down to the subcutaneous fat. With an understanding of the anatomy and physiology of the skin, it is easy to see that no agent can make its way to the fatty layer by going through the skin to get there.

If your hair is falling out from your scalp but not from your eyebrows, there is a plausible explanation based on the normal hair growth cycle. If you note that your body odor is centered under your arms and made worse by stressful events in your life, an understanding of the physiology of the sweat glands will give you the tools to figure out the cause of your problem.

You are a teenager with bad acne on your face and perfect skin on your buttocks. Why are you being punished with pimples only in areas that are in full view of your friends and everyone else in the world? An understanding of the specialized hair follicles of the face that are responsible for acne will answer the question for you.

As you read the rest of this book, there will be many other instances where an understanding of how the skin functions will give you better insights as to why things go wrong with the skin and how specific remedies can be beneficial. You may be surprised to find out that nails, hair, and sweat glands are included in this discussion. These structures are appendages of the skin; the cells that form them are derived from the same cells that make up the skin itself. Figure 2.1, shown below, is a schematic view of the skin and its appendages.

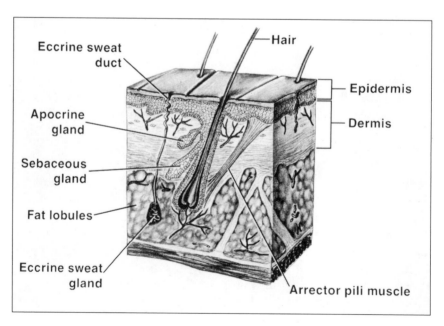

Figure 2.1   Cross-sectional representation of the skin and its appendages.

The skin is composed of two layers: the epidermis and the dermis. Below the skin is the subcutaneous fat layer. The epidermis is the paper-thin outer layer made up of several columns of cells, forming what looks like a brick wall. On the surface of the epidermis is the horny layer, the skin's outer shell.

There are no blood vessels in the epidermis. If you scrape your knee and don't injure the skin below the epidermis, you do not bleed.

Keratinocyte

The epidermis functions as a semipermeable barrier to harmful external agents. It selectively allows some substances to enter the body. It also prevents water and other crucial materials from exiting. The key component in the epidermis is the keratinocyte. It is the cell that eventually changes into the protective horny substance at the top of the skin. The keratinocyte originates at the bottom layer of the epidermis. Some cells remain there after dividing to "give birth" to new keratinocytes. These mother cells are called basal keratinocytes. Each one divides about every nineteen days; the daughter cells then begin their journey upward toward the surface. During the fourteen days that it takes to migrate to the highest level, the cells undergo many carefully programmed changes. By the time they reach the top of the epidermis, the cells bear no resemblance to their appearance just after their creation. They are flat and composed of a rigid protein called keratin, and they cover the top of the skin as the horny layer. This is the coating that the skin uses to protect itself. It is surrounded by oily membranes that insulate it from the outside world. Once in place, the horny layer remains intact for about fourteen days, when new horny layer cells move up to replace old ones. When you shower, fine brown scales come off your skin. You have probably viewed them as dirt that was being dislodged by vigorous scrubbing. Actually, it is the old horny layer that is being shed. If you have ever worn a cast for a few weeks, you may have noticed that when it was removed there were thick scales on your skin. This was the horny layer that could not wear off normally; instead, it piled up on itself.

There are a few areas of the skin that do not produce horny cells. These are the mucous membranes that line the mouth, the vagina, the tip of the penis, and the inner surface of the eyelids. These specialized structures produce no scales, which would be quite a nuisance in your eye, for example. Instead, the cells shrink as they approach the surface and peel off without forming a horny layer.

In many cases, the scaliness that you see on your skin is interpreted as dry skin. Often, this scale does not represent dryness, but rather adherent horny layer cells. The skin condition called icthyosis is an example. The horny cells do not shed in a timely fashion, leading to an accumulation of thick scales.

The horny layer is an excellent barrier against water loss and external assaults. As you get older, this barrier becomes more porous. Many older people develop dry skin because the keratinocytes are not as active as they were during youth. They make a thinner and less effective horny layer, which leads to increased water loss through the skin.

The keratinocytes can produce too much horny layer in certain disease states. In psoriasis, for example, the basal layer keratinocytes divide every thirty-six hours instead of every nineteen days. This results in a markedly thickened horny layer because the cells pile up on one another, which leads to the characteristic scaly spots of psoriasis.

Melanocyte

Wedged between the keratinocytes at the base of the epidermis are the pigment-producing cells, the melanocytes. There is approximately one melanocyte for every ten basal layer keratinocytes. During fetal life, these cells arise in the developing nervous system and move into the skin. Thus, a melanocyte has more in common with a nerve cell than with a keratinocyte. Even its appearance is more characteristic of a cell in the nervous system. It has a central body and several arm-like projections (dendrites) that communicate with the surrounding keratinocytes.

The melanocyte has one function: to produce and distribute pigment to the surrounding keratinocytes. The pigment is manufactured in an organelle in the center of the melanocyte called the melanosome. A complex protein, melanin, is made and then transported through the dendrites of the melanocyte to many of the nearby keratinocytes. These cells carry the pigment up with them into the horny layer where they are shed. There are two forms of melanin, each with a different hue. Eumelanin is dark brown, and pheomelanin has a reddish tint. All melanocytes have the capacity to make both forms of melanin.

Why does one person have dark brown skin, while another has ruddy skin, and still another has an almost milk-white complexion? Skin color depends on one's genetic makeup. African Americans have more melanocytes that produce more melanin. Most of this is the dark eumelanin variety. The melanocytes are packaged in the melanosomes singly and are distributed throughout the epidermis. Whites have fewer melanocytes and those they have make less melanin than those in black skin. The melanosomes package the melanin in tight bundles and distribute them less widely than in black skin. For these reasons, whites are lighter in color than blacks. Individuals with a ruddy complexion have melanocytes that make more of the red pheomelanin, which accounts for the reddish color in their skin.

Melanin has chemical properties that allow it to absorb and "de-energize" ultraviolet light so that it is no longer harmful. The more melanin you have in your skin, the better the protection it affords you. This only holds true for eumelanin. The red pheomelanin is not very good at blocking ultraviolet light. This is why redheads tend to sunburn much more easily than those with darker skin. Sunlight and sun protection are covered in more detail in chapter 4.

Pigmentation varies over different parts of our bodies because there are differences in melanocyte density. The face has many melanocytes and is often a little darker than other body areas. It also tans better because there are more melanocytes to be stimulated by the sun. This is evident in the light-colored palms of African-Americans

The skin changes color as people age. At age fifteen, you had the energy to run ten miles; your muscles were young and able. At age sixty, the will is there but the physical stamina is not. It is very difficult to run long distances because, even if you stay in top shape, there are anatomic changes in your muscles that make them less efficient. The melanocytes are no different. As people get older, they make less melanin and the skin lightens, whether they are white, Asian, or black. This does not always happen uniformly. Confetti-like areas of decreased pigment are commonly noted on the legs and forearms. This condition is given a big name that will keep you off guard. It is called idiopathic guttate hypomelanosis. Think of it as the skin's equivalent of graying hair.

As mentioned earlier, melanocytes share many similarities with nerve cells. When the nervous system is injured, the cells have a quite limited capacity to renew themselves; therefore the injuries have permanent consequences. When melanocytes are injured or destroyed, it is difficult for the skin to repopulate itself with new pigment-producing cells (although there is some limited potential for cells from hair follicles to migrate into the epidermis). After skin injuries such as burns or scrapes, the resulting scar is often lighter in color than the normal skin. This is because melanocytes have been destroyed, and now that part of the skin lacks the machinery to make melanin.

There are times when the skin heals with a darker color than normal after an injury. This is not because the melanocytes have juiced up their melanin production. Rather, the injury has caused melanin to fall into the deeper portion of the skin where it is engulfed by scavenger cells that hold it permanently for safe keeping. It cannot move up and be discharged from the surface since it is in cells that do not have that capacity, so it remains there indefinitely.

Sweat Glands

One of the most important functions of the skin is to regulate core body temperature. This is accomplished by two means: blood flow through the skin and evaporation of sweat secreted onto the skin's surface. There are two types of sweat glands—eccrine and apocrine. The eccrine glands produce the sweat that pours out of us when we get overheated. The apocrine glands produce a milky substance that has no useful function, other than to give a locker room its distinctive odor.

There are at least two million eccrine sweat glands located over almost all of the body surface. They are not present on the mucous membranes. (Sweat originating in the eyes would be a terrible development. It is bad enough when sweat drips into the eyes from the forehead.) These glands are composed of a secretory portion where sweat is formed and a duct that leads from the gland to the outside through a minute pore in the skin surface.

Sweat is composed mainly of water. Salt, proteins, and other trace elements are also present. Many medications are excreted through the sweat. Sweat can also be used as the vehicle to deliver an effective therapy to the skin, as is discussed later in the section on fungal infections.

Perspiration is controlled by a sweat center in the brain. As blood flows through this center, an elevated temperature of the plasma stimulates a nerve impulse to be sent to the sweat glands, which signals them to create and secrete sweat. As the sweat evaporates, the blood flowing through the skin cools. This cooler blood travels back to the sweat center and shuts off the impulse to produce more sweat. In dry climates, this physiologic evaporative cooler works very efficiently. When it is humid, however, water on the skin evaporates poorly and the body temperature may remain elevated for prolonged periods. This leads to the fatigued feeling that we all have when trying to survive a humid day in the summer.

Sweat rates vary greatly among individuals. Men usually sweat more than women. Those who are in good physical condition and perspire regularly during workouts tend to sweat sooner and more profusely when the body temperature rises. It is almost as if the sweat glands are rounded into shape as you improve your cardiovascular condition. Sweating varies in different body sites in the same person. The palms have more sweat glands than the back and produce more sweat. With age, the sweat glands function less efficiently. Older people may have less heat tolerance because they cannot keep the body sufficiently cool by sweating.

Sweating is under central nervous system control and responds to stress-driven stimuli as well as to heat. We have all experienced sweaty palms when under duress. Anyone with a teenager out alone with the family car knows exactly what I mean.

The body's other type of sweat gland is the apocrine gland. It has a limited distribution under the arms, on the nipples, in the groin area, and on the eyelids. These glands consist of a portion deep in the skin that makes the fluid and a duct that delivers it into the hair follicle. It does not have a separate pore to the outside like the eccrine gland. Apocrine sweat is a turbid, odorless fluid that is broken down by bacteria on the skin to an odoriferous substance. When one talks about body odor, apocrine sweat is the major culprit. (For a detailed discussion of body odor, see the section on antiperspirants in chapter 3.)

Does apocrine sweat serve any useful purpose in humans? Aside from stimulating a thriving antiperspirant industry, there is none of which I am aware. In dogs and other animals, modified apocrine gland secretions serve as sex attractants. This is the reason that they are constantly sniffing each other's posteriors. Humans have evolved to display their sexual wares by other means. The apocrine glands remain as a reminder of what our distant ancestors had to go through to get a date.

Hair Follicles

Hairs are derived from special epidermal cells, something like the cells that produce the horny layer of the skin. The follicle is the site where the hair is produced. There are 80,000 to 120,000 follicles on the scalp, all of which are present at birth. Most newborns are nearly bald because the hairs are fine and almost invisible. The hair shaft is made of keratin protein similar to that of the horny layer of the skin. It is lubricated with an oily substance secreted by the sebaceous gland which opens into the follicle. There is a muscle attached to the follicle that causes the hair to stand on end or to produce goose bumps. There is no reason for us to possess the capacity to do this; our evolutionary forebears may have needed this maneuver to look more ferocious to predators. But goose bumps don't look that scary on humans.

The hair is manufactured in the depths of the follicle by matrix cells, much like the basal keratinocytes. Once the hair becomes keratin, it is essentially dead. You cannot repair damaged hair or bring it back to life. Nothing you do to the ends of the hair affects the growth rate or any other metabolic behavior of the live portion of the hair. Cutting or shaving the hair has no effect whatever on the rate of growth of the new hair.

All hair has some color, at least until middle age, when the follicular melanocytes stop functioning at full capacity. Melanocytes at the base of the follicle add melanin pigment to the growing shaft, and it is carried to the surface with the emerging hair. The exact hue depends on the mixture of different melanin types and the number of active pigment cells; this is genetically determined.

There are two types of hair: vellus and terminal. Vellus hairs are the fine, downy, lightly pigmented hairs that babies have all over their bodies. When people go bald, the hair follicles don't disappear. They stop making thick hairs and start producing vellus hairs instead. Terminal hairs are the coarse hairs that are on the scalp, in the underarm area, in the pubic region, and on the extremities. Some people are naturally more hirsute than others. This is a family trait in certain racial groups. There is nothing that you can do to change this pattern of hair growth. In chapter 3, I discuss ways to remove unwanted hair.

Hair growth is under hormonal control. At puberty the male hormones (androgens), present in both men and women, stimulate the hair follicles that are making vellus hairs to begin the production of the coarser and darker terminal hairs. Pubescent children begin to have pubic and axillary hair because of increased androgen production.

All hairs have a set cycle that consists of growth, resting, shedding, and regrowth of new hair. There is a growth (anagen) phase during which the hair grows at a rate of about 0.3 to 0.4 millimeters per day. After a variable time, the hair enters a transitional (catagen) phase, which leads to a resting phase (telogen). When a new growth phase begins, a new hair is produced and the old resting hair is shed. These are the hairs you see at bottom of the shower after you shampoo. Don't worry that you were too rough in cleansing your scalp and this caused the hair to fall out. The ones that came out were being pushed from below by new hairs, rather than being yanked by you from above. Most people lose about one hundred hairs per day from the scalp.

The longer the anagen phase, the longer the hair will ultimately be. For those lucky few with growth phases lasting years, hair down to the waist is possible. Hair growth phases vary by age and location. As we get older, the anagen phase of scalp hairs gets shorter and the telogen phase lengthens. If you find that your hair is not growing as long as it used to do in your youth, it is probably because the growth phase has shortened. The scalp follicles slowly wither over time as well. Ultimately, follicles that produced vigorous terminal hairs now make only fine vellus hairs. These are not easily used to cover that persistent bald spot over the crown of your scalp.

If all the hairs on our body grew continuously for years at a time, we would bear a close resemblance to our chimpanzee cousins. We look different from chimps because of the variable length of the growth phase in different body sites. Our eyebrow hair does not grow across our face because these hairs are programmed to have a long resting phase and a relatively short growth phase. It is for this reason that it is unwise to shave your eyebrows unless you wish to be without them for a long time.

For most of one's life, hairs cycle randomly; some are in the resting phase and others are in the growth phase. Occasionally, many of the hairs synchronously enter the resting phase and then shed as a new growth cycle begins. This is called telogen effluvium. The most common time this happens is after one gives birth. Near the end of pregnancy, a large percentage of the scalp hairs go into the resting phase. A few months after delivery, the hairs resume the growth phase together, and the old hairs fall out in large clumps. In a sense, the hair fall is good news because it means that new healthy hairs are on the way. That is a little difficult to explain to an anxious patient who presents me with a bag full of hair removed from the shower basin after a single shampoo. Telogen effluvium may also occur several months after a serious illness. If your hair mysteriously begins to fall out, count back three to six months to see if you were sick or underwent an operation about that time. Severe emotional trauma can do the same thing.

Nails

Nails have evolved in lower animals and in humans because they serve important functions. They protect the end of the finger and are indispensable in grasping and holding objects. Another obscure but important function of nails is scratching. This may sound a bit farfetched, but not only does scratching feel good, it can also remove from the skin potentially harmful substances that provoke itching.

Like hair, nails are derived from the same kind of cells that produce the horny layer of the skin, and they are both made of keratin protein. Nails grow out from an area called the matrix, which lies beneath the base of the nail. The half-moon structure (lunula) that you see beneath the nail is also a part of this growth center. The nail unit is made up of the nail plate, what is generally referred to as the nail.

Below the nail plate is the nail bed, which contains fragile tissue, including many blood vessels. A wayward hammer blow to the top of the finger demonstrates well how easy it is to cause bleeding from these blood vessels. The nail plate protects this area from trauma. The cuticle is a thin layer of cells that extends from the base of the nail onto the top of the nail plate.

Unlike hair, there is no resting phase of nail growth and no spontaneous shedding. Growth is continuous throughout life. Fingernails grow about 0.1 millimeter per day, and toenails grow only one third as fast as fingernails. It takes about six months for an average fingernail to grow out completely; a toenail takes about eighteen months. Nail growth slows down during serious illnesses and as people get older.

Nail plate keratin is dead protein. There is no way to bring it back to life. Since it is exposed to the elements for months before growing to the end of the digit, it often looks very used. This normal wear and tear is unavoidable and does not affect subsequent nail growth. If you are in a hurry to get an ugly nail to grow out and be replaced by a new beautiful one, be patient. There is nothing you can do to alter the nail growth process. If you really hate the way your nails appear, try some of the approaches described in chapter 7.

Dermis

Whereas the epidermis functions as a barrier against the outside, the dermis is the support structure that anchors and nourishes the epidermis. It is composed of tough proteins that continually remodel the skin to give it its tough constitution. Collagen is the main structural protein in the dermis. It is formed in cells called fibroblasts and is deposited as incredibly strong fibers. The firm feel that you sense when you pinch the skin is due to the collagen.

The other structural protein in the dermis is elastin. Its structure is much less rigid than that of collagen, so it can deform and return to its original shape. When you pinch your skin and it returns to its original position, the elastic property of elastin in the dermis is at work.

The amorphous material that surrounds collagen and elastin is the ground substance. It holds water that keeps the dermis from drying out. It also acts as a buffer to protect the structural proteins.

The skin has far more blood vessels than it needs to nourish itself. Complex networks of small arteries and veins act as radiators to dissipate excess heat. After a strenuous workout in a hot environment, you may be beet red. This is because the heat receptor in the central nervous system senses that your body is overheating and sends out an impulse to the blood vessels in the skin. This signal causes the vessels to open up as widely as possible so that more blood can flow near the surface. As the blood circulates this way, it is cooled by the outside air and leads to core body cooling. You look flushed because there is more red blood near the surface. Likewise, on very cold days, the heat receptor closes down the blood supply to the skin so that heat can be conserved. This is particularly evident in your hands, which look very pale on a cold winter's morning.

The dermis is supplied with many nerves that signal your brain about the outside environment. Light touch is perceived because of the nerves that permeate the skin. Pain perception is also transmitted from these superficial nerves. Without these warning signals, your body could be seriously damaged before you could respond. There are several diseases in which that is exactly what happens. People with advanced diabetes mellitus lose sensation, particularly on the feet. Something as trivial as a friction blister often goes unnoticed until it has turned into an ulceration that may never heal. Leprosy is a bacterial infection that destroys the cutaneous nerves. Those unfortunate individuals with this malady lose fingers and toes because they do not have any sensation in those areas and injure them to the point where the digits literally fall off. The lesson to be learned is, don't curse when you touch a hot stove. The pain you feel is a warning from the nerves in your skin to your brain to move your hand in a hurry.

3

Skin Care Basics

No organ of the body (other than the liver in hard-drinking people) is more abused than the skin and its appendages, the hair and nails. The skin shares a border with a cruel world, which damages, dries, and ages it. The hair and nails are also constantly battered by the forces of the environment. There are times when we are a large part of the problem in our efforts to look younger, sexier, trendier, and just plain different from the way that nature intended. Luckily, there are plenty of simple things that we can do to minimize these problems. In this chapter, routine skin, hair, and nail care will be discussed, easy-to-follow programs will be described, and many myths will be dispelled.

Before discussing a specific skin care program, some general principles of identifying the best products need to be addressed. The advertising industry has been effective at creating demand for all kinds of cure-alls because claims of "scientific data" appeal to guilt about less-than-perfect looks, to the "younger-is-better" philosophy of life, to "environmental" concerns, and to protection from the polluting influences of "chemicals." How do these claims stand up to closer scrutiny? Let us review a number of the claims and beauty notions promoted by the cosmetic industry and then develop some general recommendations. We will start by discussing buzzwords that you will encounter.

Natural. When you think of natural things, images of quiet brooks, changing leaves on the trees, and pure mountain snows come to mind. You also see pure, unadulterated, healthful images. That sounds great, but what does that have to do with skin care products?

First, there is no FDA definition for "natural." Although you would expect that the source of the ingredients is from nature, be it botanical, mineral, or animal, it can also mean that the product imitates nature or is a precursor of some natural substances that are in the human body. A product can describe itself as natural even if one percent of its ingredients qualify as a natural product. Second, the idea that somehow chemicals are bad for you is ridiculous. The vast majority of synthetic agents in cosmetics or other products are harmless, and in many cases they are critical to the safety and effectiveness of the product. For example, if preservatives were not placed in most cosmetics, they would spoil or become contaminated with infectious agents. Even so-called natural preservatives such as vitamin E are organic compounds with chemical structures similar to those synthesized in the laboratory.

Just because something comes from nature does not necessarily mean that it will be of benefit. I would not go out of my way to rub poison ivy on my skin to get the soothing feeling of cool leaves. Natural products are by no means more effective than comparable synthetic agents. Also, since many natural products come directly from the wild, it is quite possible that there will be differences from batch to batch of the same product.

Hypoallergenic. This term suggests that the product is less likely to produce an allergic reaction, although the manufacturers rarely tell us against which "allergenic" product this is compared. The whole issue of allergies to skin care agents is grossly overrated. This is not a serious problem. The vast majority of reactions to topically applied products are irritant rather than allergic. Hypoallergenic agents are not necessarily any more protective against these irritant reactions, or any kinder to your skin.

Anti-aging. Ah, to be young again. To have skin as smooth as a baby's backside. What would you pay to have this become a reality? Apparently, the masses are paying millions in this quest. What are these products, and if they are so special why haven't they been placed in the water supply yet? Most of these agents contain sunscreens, which, if used chronically, can reduce sun-induced aging changes in the skin (See chapter 4). Sunscreens are a good idea, but often there is a low sun protection factor (SPF) in these cosmetics. It would make a lot more sense to choose a separate sunscreen with a high SPF if you are serious about protecting your skin from the sun. Some new moisturizers have been formulated to include high SPF sunscreens, and these are worth using. Retin-A and alpha hydroxy acids may actually reverse aging skin changes. These will be discussed in detail later in this chapter.

pH balanced. A notion that has been embraced by the cosmetic industry is that there is an optimal degree of acidity (pH) for the skin, and the closer you get to this magic number, the better your skin will look and feel. The problem is that the more alkaline (higher pH) cleansers and shampoos function better. However, higher pH products tend to be more irritating to the skin and more damaging to the hair. You must decide whether you want better cleansing or a milder product. It is hard to achieve both simultaneously.

Environmental protectant. There are many bad things that can happen to your body when you live in a big, dirty city, but pollution of your skin is not one of them. There is absolutely no evidence that city dwellers have less healthy skin than those who live in the country. Airborne grit is not your skin's mortal enemy. When products claim to offer this type of protection, they often contain a sunscreen, an antioxidant such as vitamin E or vitamin C, or both. More about these additives later, but there is little reason to select a product for this reason alone.

Dermatologist-tested. This demonstrates the classic appeal to authority, one that is highly effective in giving a product respectability. This could mean that dermatologists conducted independent tests and have delivered unbiased results to the manufacturer. If the dermatologists conclude that the product is not fit for human use, the company could still promote it as having been tested by experts without informing you, the consumer, about the results of the tests. We dermatologists are bombarded by free samples of new products and are asked to rate them on what our office receptionist or mother-in-law thinks of them. Does this qualify as "dermatologist-tested"? The answer is yes.

Microtargeted, nourishing hydrobeads, etc. Cosmetic science has progressed greatly over the past decade. New and exciting discoveries have led to elegant products. However, because a product contains what sounds like a fancy new ingredient does not automatically qualify it for the cosmetic hall of fame. Be skeptical of claims of great scientific breakthroughs.

Besides specific types of advertisements to be wary of, there are a number of general truisms that I would like to propose. I will tell you in advance that some of these reflect my skeptical nature. You may be more of a believer than I am:

- Avoid products that make statements in which benefits are based on the fact that changes "seem" to occur. For example, many products claim that they make wrinkles seem to disappear, or they calm fine lines, or they affect the appearance of your skin.

What they are telling you is that there is no real change in your skin, although your appearance may improve. This is a reasonable reason to buy a product. It just bothers me that the advertisers don't come out and say this.

- Don't listen when they substitute hyperbole for a genuine discussion of what the product does. For example, a manufacturer might claim that its moisturizer leaves your skin "deeply purified, visibly toned, and enriched." What does that mean? They could easily be discussing one's feeling after a Yanni concert.

- Don't believe them when they say their cosmetic "penetrates deeply." Although there are exceptions to the rule, the molecules of most compounds are too large to be absorbed deep into the skin. This is actually a good thing since there are many blood vessels in the upper dermis (see chapter 2), which will quickly carry compounds that are meant to stay on the skin's surface into the general circulation.

- If a product claims to have been developed at a spa in Eastern Europe by a famous chemist, hold onto your wallet. Almost without exception, these types of skin care products are expensive, contain unusual but useless ingredients, and offer nothing better than what the cosmetic scientists in the good ol' USA can deliver.

- If the product claims to do anything whatever to your pores, think twice before buying it. Pores are the openings through which hairs emerge and lubricating oil (sebum) is secreted. They may be prominent, but there is little that one can do to change this. You can't close your pores. They don't have little muscles that can contract if given the appropriate stimulus. If you use a cleanser some of the retained oil or dirt can be removed from the pores, but there are few agents that do this much better than soap and water.

- The efficacy of a skin care program is not directly proportional to what you pay for it. Some of the best products can be purchased in drugstores or supermarkets at one tenth the cost of brands sold in spas or department stores. A beautiful bottle or package can contain a mediocre cosmetic. Don't get caught in the trap of measuring your self-image by how exotic the product line that you buy is. In fact, many products sold by the most exclusive cosmetic houses are identical to those sold by generic retailers and are manufactured in the same factories with the same formulas.

The high-priced products do have nice containers and are sold by well-clad salespeople, however.

- You do not need to buy the entire product line to benefit from individual agents. A corollary to this is that you don't necessarily need a different preparation for different skin sites. Select only those items that suit your individual needs.

- If any claims are made about an item improving your "cellulite problem," don't buy the product. This entire cellulite business is invented by those who wish to give us another reason to feel bad about normal fat beneath our skin. In some people these fatty deposits are distributed in such a way as to produce a dimpling effect. There is no way that these deposits can be altered by any manipulation from the skin's surface.

- Don't trust a cosmetic that claims to rejuvenate, relieve, strengthen, repair, nourish, purify, rebuild, or diminish some defect in your skin. By definition, cosmetics can have no permanent effects on your skin. Drugs are defined as agents that affect the structure or function of the human body. If the manufacturers of these cosmetics are obeying FDA regulations, they are not being quite so forthcoming with you, the consumer. It is not the responsibility of the marketers of these cosmetics to portray their products in other than the most glowing terms. It is your responsibility to be realistic and hard-nosed when it comes to evaluating these agents.

- Don't assume that because some beautiful movie star endorses a skin care product, it alone is the reason for that person's good looks and success. Genetics and a skilled plastic surgeon may have also contributed something to the spectacular result.

- Facial exercises or "workouts" don't prevent the skin's aging process. Don't pay thousands of dollars to an expert in the field so that you can find this out firsthand. Wrinkles do not occur because of faulty muscle tone in the face. Facial muscle movements can deepen expression lines. The purveyors of this approach claim that by exercising these muscles, one increases the "health" of the muscles and stimulates collagen and elastin deposition in the overlying skin, a proposition that I find impossible to believe.

After reading this introduction, you might think that it is a hopeless cause finding the appropriate approach to your skin care needs.

Actually, it is not a difficult task. There are many outstanding products to choose from. Once you understand some basic concepts about your skin and what it requires and determine what your individual needs and preferences are, your skin will look great and you will feel better about yourself. For the rest of this chapter, we will discuss basic skin hygiene. This includes cleansing and moisturizing, skin tune-ups with exfoliators (some of which may double as wrinkle creams), sweating, body odor, and care of hair and nails. First, we will address the contentious issue of nutrition and how it might affect your skin.

Nutrition and the Skin

Two common questions posed to me by my patients are whether certain nutritional deficiencies are causing their skin problem and whether nutritional additives will affect how their skin looks. The concept of the connection between food and general health is not a new one. A famous nutritionist once stated that, "You are what you eat." I suspect she never saw all the junk food-eating children with beautiful skin that we all know and love.

Your body works like a finely tuned machine that incorporates what it needs and stores or excretes anything left over. It does not need certain foods to thrive, but certain *nutrients* are necessary regardless of the form they take. If you have taken the appropriate daily requirement of vitamin A, for example, mega-amounts above that are simply stored in the liver or not absorbed from the gastrointestinal tract. Your skin never sees additional quantities of this vitamin, because your system does not recognize the requirement. This principle holds true for essentially all nutrients. Therefore skin tune-ups taken at the health food stores are destined to fail.

Patients often ask me to check them for possible nutritional deficiencies, hoping that a simple adjustment in some vitamin will make them look like they did years earlier. First, in spite of the massive amounts of less-than-healthy food that we all eat, there are very few people I see who are nutritionally deficient to the point where their skin is somehow affected. It is easy to achieve the minimal nutritional goals for healthy skin. Severe vitamin deficiencies do produce profound skin and mucous membrane changes. In the developed countries of the world, this is seldom seen, particularly in patients seeking advice about their appearance. The human body is, indeed, a wonderful thing. Teenagers can live on Big Macs and fries and still remain relatively healthy. (Don't tell your teenage children this fact of life. It would ruin the lectures you have carefully constructed about nutrition and health. There will be more about this in the section on acne.)

Are there any skin conditions that can be helped by changing your diet? If you are a dog, the answer is a resounding yes. If you feed dogs a high fat diet, the oil content in their coats will increase and improve the texture and appearance. Unfortunately, we humans can't bark, scratch our ears with our hind legs, or increase the oil content in our dry skin by eating a high fat diet. Likewise, drinking large quantities of water will not increase the moisture in your skin, unless you are severely dehydrated. The kidneys keep our systemic water balance tightly regulated. If you start drinking water by the gallon to improve your dry skin condition, prepare to do so near a restroom, since all excess water will soon be excreted.

Skin Cleansing

All of us would agree that an essential part of good hygiene is keeping the skin as clean as possible. However, too much of a good thing can cause problems. It is important to put the goal of clean skin in the perspective of what it accomplishes for you and what price you pay to achieve it. Intertwined in this discussion is the notion of "skin type." This idea has made what could be a simple issue into one where computers are integrating a great deal of data to tell you about the unique qualities of your skin, almost like your personal fingerprint. A person's skin is not a static anatomic and functional unit. It changes with age, weather, menstrual cycles, emotions, makeup, and other skin care products. Almost all of us have regional variations in the character of our skin. For example, the central part of the face contains more oil glands that make the skin a little bumpier and oilier than at the sides of the cheeks and forehead. Therefore, most of us would have what has been labeled "combination skin." To call this a special skin type only complicates our lives unnecessarily.

It is important to realize that there is no standard "perfect" skin that we all must strive to emulate. If your skin is somewhat on the dry side and you don't mind, live and be well with it. Likewise, if washing once daily satisfies your needs for adequate hygiene, there is no compelling reason to wash more often. Sorry folks, but cleanliness is not next to godliness when it comes to your skin. Many compulsive washers damage their skin by frequent cleansing. Therefore, for the remainder of this discussion, I am going to emphasize the notion of being as gentle to your skin as possible while achieving good hygiene.

There are several alternatives to choose from for washing the face and body. The three categories of cleansers are soaps, water-soluble creams or lotions, and wipe-off cleansers, which are mainly used to remove makeup. Most people use bar soaps with water because they work well at removing surface dirt, sweat, oil, cosmetics, and bacteria. If your face is oily, one of the antibacterial soaps, which are somewhat drying, would be your best choice. Although most people have little problem with irritation from the ingredients in these products, you may have a little better luck with unscented varieties. If you have acne, this type of soap is probably best for you unless your anti-acne medications have already dried out your face excessively. You will find a complete discussion of acne in chapter 5.

If your skin is dry or sensitive to ordinary bar soap, you have many good alternatives. Superfatted soaps contain additional fatty materials such as cold cream, cocoa butter, or lanolin, which make them less drying. However, you sacrifice some cleansing power with these preparations. Transparent soaps contain more fat and glycerin, which are easier on dry skin. However, these products don't lather very well and have an annoying habit of melting away in the bath or shower, so they don't last as long as milled soap. Many additives are placed in soap bars that supposedly improve the skin, such as aloe, vitamins, vegetables, fruits, herbs, and special oils. There is no way that you can nourish the skin from the surface. Avoid products with these extraneous additives. In a recent study published in a leading consumer magazine, twenty-five soaps were assessed for mildness. Dove, one of the least expensive brands, was the winner.

Water-soluble cleansers are a good choice for those with sensitive skin. These do not cleanse quite as well as bar soaps and most don't provide you with a rich lather, but they do remove surface dirt and makeup. To use this product, wet your face with water, then gently rub in the cleanser, preferably without a washcloth (to minimize the irritation of rubbing). There are many brands ranging in price from six to fifty dollars per bottle. Two inexpensive and effective cleansers of this type are Cetaphil lotion and Aquanil lotion. Both of these products are unscented and very gentle. Several new foams or gel cleansers have been introduced to the market. These lather well but can leave your skin dry. They tend to be quite costly. Cold cream is still one of the most widely used cleansing agents, particularly to remove makeup and surface debris. It tends to be heavier than the water-soluble lotions; therefore, it produces a drag on the skin when being applied and is more difficult to remove.

For those of you with an oily complexion, a more vigorous cleansing regimen may be needed. Drying antibacterial soaps provide a cheap and easy way to reduce oils. Premoistened cleansing pads, often with alcohol as a major ingredient, are also useful. Abrasive soaps might be tempting to use because they are "strong," but you really don't want to substitute inflamed skin for an oily complexion. Other approaches to an oily complexion will be discussed later in this chapter. Another convenient means of removing excess oil from the face is to use absorbent papers, which are sold in pharmacies or at cosmetic counters. Simply blot your face with these sheets, and the oil will be absorbed onto the paper.

Moisturizing Agents

Aside from soap, moisturizers are probably the most important preparation that you can apply to your skin if, and only if, you have dry skin. I say this because moisturizers accomplish exactly one thing: they retain moisture in the skin so that the surface is smooth and not scaly. The following is a partial list of what moisturizers do not do:

- get rid of wrinkles.

- prevent wrinkling or other signs of skin aging.

- add nutrients to the skin.

- promote cellular regeneration.

Dry skin (xerosis) occurs in many people as they age because the skin loses some capacity to hold water. Most people will have at least some evidence of dry skin during long, cold winters because the combination of the cold outside temperatures and the low humidity that occurs in houses with forced-air heating causes increased evaporation from the skin. In my part of the country, nearly everyone suffers from dryness to some extent. In Florida, this is far less common because of the high humidity. Frequent bathing, swimming, or showering can remove the protective oils that help to keep your skin moist and can lead to further drying.

How do you know if you have dry skin? This is a functional definition. There is increased water loss through the skin, which can be quantified by sophisticated experimental techniques. Since it is unlikely that your next birthday present will be an evaporimeter, you must rely on subtle signs and symptoms of xerosis. Dry skin may be scaly and has a rough feel but not all scaly conditions are "dry" conditions. For example, seborrhea is a disease with very scaly and greasy areas. Patients with this problem do not have dry skin; they are just making scale too fast for the body to remove it efficiently. Many with dry skin are itchy, particularly after bathing. Xerosis is by far the most common cause of itchiness without a rash. If your skin is itchy for no obvious reason, try a moisturizer before running to the dermatologist.

There are two ways that moisturizers, also known as emollients or lubricants, work to improve your skin. One is to prevent the dry air from absorbing the water from the skin. If the air is dry, there is almost a wick effect in the skin where water is drawn up to the surface and then evaporates. The other thing that moisturizers accomplish is to hold water in the skin. Although all lubricants contain water, they do not add this moisture to the skin. Most of the water in moisturizers evaporates shortly after application, leaving behind a layer of protective oil, which performs the task of lubricating the surface.

Moisturizing products are formulated as either oil-in-water (O/W) emulsions or water-in-oil (W/O) emulsions. W/O products are oilier, heavier, and stay on better. However, the greasy feel of many of these products is not for everyone. O/W emulsions are lighter, less greasy, and more pleasant to apply but they rub off more easily than W/O products. Preservatives are also necessary because all water-based products can be contaminated by bacteria. There are four types of oils in moisturizers. Each has slightly different properties but similar effects:

- Vegetable oils of many different types of are incorporated into emollients, from common soybean and coconut oil to exotic sandalwood, avocado, and macadamia oil. Just because an oil is imported from the South Pacific does not automatically qualify it as something special for your skin.

- Animal fats have been an integral part of moisturizers for decades because they are inexpensive and easily available. Lanolin is an example of this type of agent. It closely resembles the oil produced by human sebaceous glands.

- Mineral oils derived from petroleum, such as Vaseline, are effective and inexpensive. These have large molecules that stay on the skin surface to provide an excellent barrier. Some acne-prone individuals may have flare-ups if petroleum-based products are used on the face.

- Vitamin E is incorporated into moisturizers not for its nutrient properties but because it is an effective oil. Marketers of these products would like you to believe that the vitamin E in their products could act as a free-radical scavenger with anticancer properties. Until further notice, don't believe them. (More about this later.) Vitamin E does have one bad habit. It can cause allergic contact dermatitis. If you break out in a rash after using this agent, it could be the culprit.

For those who cannot tolerate oils in lubricants, a class of "oil-free" products has emerged. There is no strict definition or industry standard for these kinds of formulations. Most contain silicones, which are non-greasy yet have a smooth feel. Water-in-silicone emulsions feel less tacky on the skin but tend to separate in spite of emulsifier additives, so they often need to be shaken before being applied. These are the same class of chemicals that were in breast implants and caused some medical problems. When applied to the skin, however, silicones are harmless. Many of these agents are recommended for people with acne, but it is still unsettled whether they make pre-existing acne worse.

In the pursuit of your business, cosmetic chemists have developed an incredible array of additives to moisturizers. Here is a rundown on some of the more popular items.

Collagen and elastin. These proteins are an essential part of normal skin. They provide the structure that gives it its integrity. They are also hydrophilic, which means that they hold water well. That may sound like a good feature but recall that moisturizers do not add water to the skin; they simply prevent it from escaping. Marketers of these products would like us to believe that collagen and elastin somehow penetrate into the skin and improve the overall skin structure and integrity. Unfortunately, these molecules are much too large to get through the skin.

Mucopolysaccharides. These are natural components of the skin that surround the collagen and elastin and give the skin structural integrity. They also hold water, which is why they are incorporated into emollients. I wouldn't pay extra for this additive.

Miscellaneous protein extracts. If you ever want to know where the unwanted organs from the butcher go, you might check in some of the world's most fashionable beauty spas. Here you will find concoctions containing placenta, spleen, brain (neural lipid extract), thymus, blood components (serum albumin), and tendon. In an effort to clean the sea of potentially harmful algae, these dead organisms have been removed from the oceans and placed in moisturizers as sea algae extract. The person who has everything can purchase a lubricating cream containing essence of skin caviar. Here is another basic principle that you will see only in this book: Don't buy a skin care product if you can trace the origin of any of the ingredients to something that you can identify in the zoo, on the farm, or at the meat counter of the supermarket.

Vitamin A. One of the more pernicious additives being used in moisturizers today is vitamin A or one of its derivatives. Aside from being of no benefit in preventing water loss, I can't help believing that its sole purpose in being added to the formulation is to capitalize on the Retin-A fad. Vitamin A is a different compound than Retin-A and has no effectiveness whatever in the treatment of wrinkles or other manifestations of sun damage.

Liposomes. Liposomes are synthetic pellets that can penetrate deeper into the skin. If oils are attached to these structures, the idea is that these oils will make their way below the skin's surface and thus resist removal. This is a great idea, but it remains to be proven that there is any special benefit of liposomes in moisturizers.

We dermatologists are often asked to suggest to patients our favorite moisturizer. Unfortunately what is best for my skin may be totally inappropriate for you. There are a few general tips that I can give you in picking and using these agents:

- For use over the whole body, lotions are easier to apply and don't stain clothing quite as much as creams. However, they may not stay on your skin as well. For localized areas such as the hands, feet, and face, creams may be a better choice because they remain in place longer.

- If you are looking for the product that is least likely to cause an allergic reaction, choose one without a fragrance since perfumes are fairly common causes of this side effect.

- No matter how heavy your emollient is, it will still rub off during the day. For this reason, all moisturizers should be applied at least twice daily. A good time to use them is after bathing or showering in the morning while your skin is slightly damp. Bedtime is another good time to use them because if your dry skin causes itching it will be more of a bother at night when you have no other focus for your senses.

- Bath oils are a poor substitute for moisturizing creams and lotions. These oils do not stay on the skin well, so you will not get only long-term coverage. In addition, they make the bath tub very slippery and can be the direct cause for some nasty falls. If you feel like spoiling yourself, try putting a cup of corn starch or one of the commercial oatmeal preparations in your bath water. It will make your skin feel good, but it won't do much for your dry skin problem. Bathing actually dries out your skin by removing the protective surface oils.

- You do not need different moisturizers for your eyes and the rest of your face. Eyelid skin is very thin and can get irritated easily, so it needs gentle handling. However, the rest of your skin needs this degree of care. Stick with one product that feels good all over your body. There are exceptions to this rule, however. If you have exceptionally dry hands and feet, for example, heavy-duty creams or even straight petroleum jelly (Vaseline) may be necessary.

For those of you who have major dry skin problems in spite of routine use of emollients, here is the regimen I would recommend:

- Bathe or shower as infrequently as possible, not more than three times per week during the winter.

- When you do bathe, use either a nondrying soap such as Dove or a water-soluble cleanser such as Cetaphil lotion. Tepid water is preferable. Don't indulge yourself with long showers or baths since they will dry you out more.

- After emerging from the bath, towel dry until you are just slightly damp, and apply a moisturizing lotion at that point.

- If your house has forced-air heating, consider purchasing a humidifier for your bedroom.

- If you are still having problems after a three-week trial of this program, consult a dermatologist. It is possible that your problem is not dry skin but rather another skin condition that causes scaling.

Exfoliators

Normal skin is constantly renewing itself by sloughing the top (horny) layer. When these cells build up, either because of overproduction or inadequate removal, they appear as scale, feel rough to the touch, or both. Removing this excess scale does nothing to stimulate normal growth from below or to remove wrinkles, but it does make the skin feel better and might make other agents such as moisturizers work better. The cosmetic industry has developed many products that are meant to aid in the removal of excess scale. Some are also cleansers and lubricants. All of these cause some degree of skin irritation since the scale must be forcibly separated from the underlying skin, so they are not appropriate for those of you with sensitive, easily irritated skin. Here is a brief rundown on some of these agents.

COSMETIC SCRUBS

Many different particulates have been added to creams or lotions to give them a rough texture and the capacity to remove scale when rubbed on the skin. You can liken this to using a Brillo pad to remove caked-on food from a pot. If you don't scrub hard enough, the grease remains; however, if you are too vigorous, you can easily scratch the surface. Even materials such as peach pit particles or sea shell powder can be extremely abrasive. Your face deserves better than the treatment you give to your cooking utensils.

ABRASIVE BRUSHES OR PADS

Space-age materials have been incorporated into pads and other implements which supposedly gently remove scale, makeup, and dirt without harming the skin itself. These are not qualitatively different from rubbing peach pit parts on your face. If you scrub too hard, you can still irritate the skin.

FACIAL MASKS

For thousands of years people looking to improve their appearance have made themselves look temporarily strange by putting all sorts of unconventional things on their faces. In the case of facial masks, they may have been on to something. There are at least five general categories of mask constituents that have different effects on the skin. Please remember that these masks can irritate sensitive skin even if ingredients are added to help those who have difficulty with harsh products:

- Wax-based masks are popular because they are applied warm, feel good on the skin, and can make one feel relaxed. They help moisturize the face temporarily, and when removed may cleanse the skin of old cells and dirt.

- Rubber and vinyl masks are easy to apply and are often used at home. They are squeezed from a tube or pouch and applied directly to the skin. After the moisture evaporates, a soothing, thin rubber film remains. When the rubber is stripped, it removes surface oil, dirt, and skin scale.

- Earth-based masks, also known as mud packs, consist of clays that can absorb oil from greasy skin. They have also been used to treat certain forms of acne, but are of minimal benefit to most people.

- Hydrocolloid masks are used by salons and at home. They are made of large-molecular-weight substances that form a paste when mixed with water. Aside from being soothing and somewhat lubricating, many additives have been incorporated into these products which are supposed to give them extra efficacy in treating all kinds of skin conditions. Avocado, honey, almond oil, vitamin E, and many other materials may give the products a certain mystique, but they probably have little effect on the skin. Still, you may feel refreshed after treating yourself to one of these facials. That's what makes these products excellent additions to your hygiene regimen.

ALPHA HYDROXY ACIDS (AHA)

Over the past few years there has been an enormous emphasis on the old technology of AHAs. The effects of these agents were probably recognized during the time of Cleopatra. She used red wine on her face to maintain her beauty. Wine contains AHAs, and it may have been the secret behind her success as one of antiquity's most attractive women. There are now over two hundred products that contain one or more of these compounds, with claims that range from mild exfoliation to wrinkle effacement to nail rejuvenation. They are present in shampoos, moisturizers, cleansers, toners, and cosmetics. At high concentration, they are used by physicians and others as superficial or mid-depth peeling agents. (See Chapter 8.) Could millions of satisfied customers be wrong about these agents? The short answer is that we don't know for sure if these products perform as they are supposed to, but there are encouraging signs that these agents might be very useful.

The alpha hydroxy acids comprise a group of organic compounds derived from diverse sources such as fruit juices (thus the name "fruit acids"), sugar cane, milk, and grapes. Exactly how these agents work on the skin is still not completely understood, but there are currently two theories that might explain the mechanism of action. They may weaken the bonds between cells and facilitate sloughing. They may also be mild irritants that stimulate the skin to renew itself faster, losing its horny layer more efficiently. Although these products appear safe and there have been relatively few customer complaints, the FDA is looking into the issue of long-term safety, since very little information has been made available.

The main use for AHAs is as a mild exfoliant. There are so many competing products out there that it is extremely difficult to choose the one appropriate for your needs. Your first consideration should be the amount of the active ingredient. Unfortunately, many brands fail to inform the public exactly how much of a given AHA is present. If less than a 5% concentration is present, there will probably be little or no effect in spite of the claims of the manufacturer. Products containing between 5% and 15% are just about right for mild exfoliation and minimal irritancy. Although the following is not an exhaustive list of AHAs, here are just a few of the currently available brands:

- Eucerin Plus (5% AHA)

- LacHydrin Five (5% AHA)

- Alpha Hydrox (8% AHA)

- Skin Smoothing Cream (8% AHA)

- Aqua Glycolic Face Cream (12% AHA)

- M.D. Formulations Facial Lotion (12% AHA)

Some physicians sell these products in their offices and may promote them as being better than ones bought in stores. There is nothing special about the AHA preparations marketed by these practitioners; I would suggest that you demur when these products are offered for sale. As I discussed in chapter 1, you should not feel intimidated because your doctor wants you to buy only his product line. It's your money. You can probably spend it more wisely in a discount drugstore rather than his office. The one advantage to buying this from your doctor is that you can determine the exact concentration of the agent, if you ask.

If you choose to shop at a specialty counter in a department store or spa and the salesperson either doesn't know or won't reveal the amount of AHA in the product, don't buy it. Definitely do not be caught in the scam that some merchandisers try when they claim that there is a secret formula that they are not at liberty to divulge. Here is another of my general rules: "Secret" formulas are never better than public formulas. If something is so great, it will be patented and protected by patent laws, so there is absolutely no reason to hide its contents from the public.

Many of these AHA products are marketed for specific areas of the body. There is little reason to buy different AHAs or different forms of the same AHA for various sites on your skin. Pick a product that feels good and has the optimal concentration, and use it wherever you need it.

Exactly who does need AHAs? If your skin feels rough and flaky, AHAs may smooth it out to a moderate degree. If you have blackheads and whiteheads from acne, regular use of these agents may slightly control this portion of your condition.

Preparations containing AHAs are easy to use. After cleansing and drying your skin, apply a thin layer of the product as you would a moisturizer. Don't scrub it in because this can lead to added irritation. Many of these agents will cause a few seconds of mild burning, particularly on the face. If this is too intense or if it lasts for a long time, you are probably using a concentration of the AHA that is too high for your skin. To minimize the burning do not use other potential irritants, such as alcohol or harsh soaps.

For the first few weeks of use, you may notice that your skin seems flakier than usual. This is the AHA doing its job. Be patient. Once this phase passes, it rarely recurs. However, if months go by and you are still plagued by the flakiness, consider different products or even abandon AHAs altogether.

Although you may be tempted to try AHAs for all sorts of skin conditions, please remember that they are mainly useful as a mild exfoliant. They do not affect the size of your pores, nor do they close pores which are widely dilated, they have little effect on wrinkles at the concentrations that you can use at home; they do not act as lubricants, although they may help your moisturizer work a little better; but the vehicles into which they are incorporated may be lubricating; they do not control oiliness.

RETIN-A

Few drugs in the past two decades have generated as much interest and controversy as Retin-A. Even after hundreds of thousands of people have used this agent as an alleged wrinkle cream, there is still no clear consensus as to its value. Before the storm of publicity engulfed Retin-A, it was well known as an effective treatment of acne. This is still its only FDA-approved use, although dermatologists have treated many other skin conditions with it.

Retin-A is a synthetic retinoid derivative of vitamin A. It possesses a number of properties that are different from the parent compound. In experiments on test animals, it causes the skin to develop a more normal pattern of keratinization. By that I mean that with Retin-A use, the skin renews itself more closely to the way it should. It also repairs sun damaged connective tissue, increases the blood vessels in the skin, and decreases the activity of the pigment-producing cells in the skin.

If these changes would consistently occur in sun-damaged human skin, we would expect major changes in the appearance and feel of the treated areas. Unfortunately, life is not that simple. For some reason, only certain people respond to this therapy, and the changes are often subtle at best. However, there are real success stories with Retin-A, particularly in those with early changes associated with chronic sun exposure. Retin-A improvement is in the eye of the beholder. A few years ago, we conducted a study to examine the effects of Retin-A in test subjects with mildly sun damaged skin. After sixteen weeks of therapy, we investigators and the patients independently rated the improvement. It was as if we were looking at different people than the patients were. In many instances, we were impressed with the results while the patient was disappointed that nothing had happened. In other cases, the patients felt that the remarkable improvement gave them a new appearance, and we thought they had the same old looks. It is this situation that makes one wary of drawing any firm conclusions about Retin-A.

Retin-A is a real drug, not just a cosmetic, and as such must be prescribed by a physician. Remember, treatment of facial wrinkles is not an approved use of this medication. In some respects this therapy is still experimental. However, it is safe to the point that one day it may be sold over the counter. How can you determine if this is the correct treatment for you? You need a hard-hearted assessment by your dermatologist, preferably one without preconceived notions about how great or how useless Retin-A is. The criteria that he should use will include the following:

- Mild to moderate changes from sun damage, including some fine wrinkles, brown splotches, leathery feel to the skin, and perhaps a few actinic keratoses. (See chapter 4 for a complete discussion of this condition.)

- Relatively few coarse, deep wrinkles.

- Minimal skin laxity.

- Skin that is resistant to irritation.

- A person who is patient and stoic, since it may take months to see any benefit.

If you and your doctor determine that Retin-A is right for you, he will probably suggest that you start out by applying the medication every other night for the first two weeks. This will give you a chance to become accustomed to it. You should expect to have some redness and peeling; this tends to go away within the first four to six weeks, as your skin gets used to this new irritant.

Retin-A should be applied at night, at least thirty minutes after you have cleansed your face. Spread a small amount evenly over the face. If you see evidence of it on your skin after application, you are using too much. (When you find out how costly Retin-A is, you will apply very small amounts to your face.) Cleansing can be accomplished with mild bar soap or water-soluble cleansers since they won't add to the irritation that you may experience. Avoid applying the medication near the corners of your nose or eyes. Since Retin-A may make you more sensitive to the sun, it is important that you use potent sunscreens when outdoors. Try to avoid cosmetic products containing alcohol, if possible. Moisturizers are often worthwhile adjunctive agents and should be applied twice daily.

After about four months, you might see modest but noticeable changes in your skin. If you and your doctor agree that not much has happened, he may increase the strength of the medication to try to coax some improvement out of this treatment. My experience has been that if a person does not realize a benefit by six months, it is time to give up on trying to turn back the clock.

Some argue that Retin-A and AHAs do the same things for your face, so why use a strong prescription drug when easy-to-use AHAs are available? I disagree with this theory; Retin-A has distinct effects that AHAs do not. It can work on wrinkles, while AHAs have minimal effects at the concentrations used by most people. Retin-A can partially fade pigmented blotches, while AHAs cannot. Finally, Retin-A may have effects deeper in your skin, while low-concentration AHAs only affect the surface. Thus, each has its own separate uses. In some individuals, both agents are used simultaneously. Of course, one would have to have very tough skin to withstand the irritant effects of both agents.

Is Retin-A the miracle of the ages? No. Will it change your appearance radically? No. Can you derive modest benefit from its use? Yes, if you have mild changes associated with chronic sun exposure, fine wrinkling, splotches, and rough skin texture.

Other Skin Care Products

The cosmetic industry has supplied us with a product for every possible whim and fancy, and has attempted to sell these as an indispensable part of our daily hygiene regimen. Here are a few such products.

Astringents. The cosmetic industry has heavily promoted these alcohol-containing products and has given them elegant names such as toners, fresheners, and clarifying lotions. All of these products share one thing—they tingle when you apply them. This is because they are mild irritants. Some also contain exfoliants such as resorcinol or salicylic acid. I suspect that these products are popular because consumers think that something really outstanding must be happening when the skin tingles. That sensation has absolutely nothing to do with anything helpful that might be going on. These products remind me a little bit of the commercial for the aftershave lotion where the actor likens the product to a "cold slap in the face," suggesting that you need a wallop to feel better. I would suggest you use astringents only if you subscribe to that philosophy of skin care.

Cosmetic water. Special water is being sold as a substitute for what comes out of your tap, with the notion that your skin deserves the best and that European spa water has to work better because it comes from far away and because it is "pure." These waters are supplied in spray bottles from which one spritzes a little of the magic liquid onto the face before applying a moisturizer. As we discussed earlier, the function of moisturizers is to keep the water already in your skin from evaporating. When you apply water on the surface, it quickly evaporates, no matter how elegant it is. Save your money and buy something more useful, like a pet rock.

Aloe vera. The aloe plant is a succulent whose leaves contain a juice that has been used for centuries as a cure-all for skin disorders, particularly for burns and traumatic wounds. There has been some scientific interest in the juice. Although almost entirely made up of water, there are proteins that have some activity, at least in experimental systems. I have heard so often from satisfied patients that the material is soothing to burned skin that I believe this claim. I have difficulty understanding why this fact should lead to its use in shampoos, cleansers, moisturizers, shaving creams, and sunscreens. Part of the reason is that this is a "natural" product, which many consumers have a weakness for. However, by the time that the juice has been purified, pasteurized, and adulterated in myriad other ways, the aloe vera is hardly natural anymore. I would not make a special trip to the store just to purchase a product containing aloe vera.

Perspiration and Body Odor

As discussed in chapter 2, sweating is a critical bodily function that helps to maintain a proper core body temperature. We certainly do not need the odor that comes with sweating, however. Why we emit a characteristic foul smell when we sweat is a complicated business, but I will give you the highlights so that you can then understand the strategies that are employed in reducing sweating and minimizing body odor.

There are two types of sweat glands. The eccrine glands produce a colorless and odorless salty fluid, and the secretion increases when your body heats up or when you have increased emotional stimuli.

There is a different type of sweat gland, called the apocrine gland, which is present in certain areas of the body such as in the underarm area, where they are most numerous, around the nipples, and in the groin. The secretion from this gland is milky, thicker than eccrine sweat, and has a distinctive odor when acted on by surface bacteria. Apocrine glands are primarily under hormonal control. Before puberty, when hormonal stimulation of these glands is minimal, few have problems with body odor. Likewise, aged people, whose hormone levels have decreased greatly from their peak levels, also have less trouble with body odor. Apocrine glands also respond to emotional stimuli such as sexual arousal, fear, and pain.

Apocrine sweat is produced in very small amounts. However, when there is copious eccrine sweat in the area, it dissolves the apocrine sweat and disperses it over a wider area. In the moist, warm areas where apocrine glands are most prevalent bacteria grow well. These bacteria degrade the organic material in the sweat into odoriferous compounds. Each individual's apocrine sweat has a slightly different makeup. Thus, people smell different depending on what comprises the apocrine gland secretion. The sites of maximal apocrine gland activity are also hair-bearing areas. Secreted sweat fixes to the hair and gives the bacteria ample time to digest it.

Many animals have these types of smells, which function as sexual attractants. People have evolved to the point that these particular types of odors are usually not much of a turn-on. The manufacture and sale of antiperspirants is a 1.8 billion dollar business. After soap and shampoo, deodorants and antiperspirants come in third as the most popular personal skin care items. Greater than 90% of adults in the United States use some kind of underarm product daily (even in these troubled times, there still is something to be thankful for).

Based on the mechanisms by which body odor develops, cosmetic chemists have tried to attack the problem in three ways: reduce apocrine secretion, reduce eccrine secretion, and decrease bacterial growth in the sites of apocrine gland activity. There are no nonsurgical ways of reducing apocrine gland activity effectively. Therefore, attention has been focused on cutting down on eccrine sweat and by creating an environment inhospitable to bacteria.

ANTIPERSPIRANTS

By far the most commonly used products for control of body odor are the antiperspirants. These work by creating an obstructive plug in the sweat duct so that sweat cannot reach the skin surface. Since the underarm contains only a small portion of the total number of sweat glands, decreased sweating in this area does not affect overall temperature control.

There are three different chemicals from which you can choose for your antiperspirant: aluminum chloride, aluminum chlorohydrate, and aluminum zinc chlorohydrate. There is no proof of the fabled link between aluminum and Alzheimer's disease. It is important that you read the labels of the products that you plan to purchase. As you will see, some will fit your needs better than others. Aluminum chloride is the most potent of these agents. It is in only a few preparations, however, because it is often quite irritating to the skin. Avoid these products unless your excess sweating is greatly interfering with your life. The most widely used of the three chemicals is aluminum chlorohydrate. It is the mildest agent but the least potent. If you have a normal amount of sweating, this should be sufficient for your needs. A few brands contain aluminum zinc chlorohydrate. These are somewhat stronger than those containing aluminum chlorohydrate, but it would be difficult to discern a major difference between the two, except for one fact. Because of potential toxic reactions with aerosolized aluminum zinc chlorohydrate, it is not available in spray form. There is no problem with the other dosage forms of this product.

Once you have chosen the type of antiperspirant, the next step is to pick a delivery system for the drug (yes, the FDA considers these agents official drugs). As a rule, roll-ons are the most potent, followed by sticks. Aerosols are the least potent and are often the most expensive. They are also an inefficient way to deliver the drug, since invariably some will run down your arm. Since these products are potential irritants, it is best to keep them as localized as possible. Sticks and roll-ons perform that function well.

Recently there has been a spate of clear products that tap into a consumer's desire for purity. You do pay a price for using these products, however. They tend to have a more tacky feel, irritation is more common, and they leave a residue that may decrease efficacy slightly. If you are into natural things, antiperspirants are probably the wrong agents for you, because we are talking about some serious chemicals. If you overcome that hurdle, there is little reason to buy a clear product. The active ingredients are identical to those in the colored agents.

To maximize the mileage that you get out of antiperspirants, there a few guidelines to follow:

- Apply the product at night before going to bed. This gives it several hours to do what it is supposed to do before the next day's sweating begins. These chemicals do not work instantaneously, so applying an antiperspirant just before a hot date is too late. Another reason to use the agents at night is that most of us shower in the morning. If you apply the antiperspirant just after showering, the residual moisture in the underarm area may dilute it or spread it away from its site of action.

- Apply the agent only in the hair-bearing area of the underarm. There are few sweat glands out of this immediate area. Why waste it?

- Avoid shaving immediately before applying your antiperspirant, since shaving will increase the potential for these already irritating substances to cause more inflammation under your arms.

- These products have long-lasting effects. They may keep you dry for at least a full day, if not longer. Therefore, there is no compelling reason to apply them more than once daily. You probably could get away with four or five applications per week.

DEODORANTS

Unlike antiperspirants, deodorants control body odor without any effect on sweating. Most deodorants work by masking the odor of the sweat with a competing, and presumably nicer, smell. There are a few products that contain an antibacterial agent, which controls odor by minimizing the bacteria that break down sweat. Since most antiperspirants contain a fragrance as well, there is almost no reason to rely on pure deodorants unless you are one of the few individuals who reacts to all three chemicals that are in antiperspirants. Before placing the blame on the active ingredients, try different formulations. I personally have never seen a reaction to one of the stick products, so try one or two of those first.

There are some additional measures that can maximize the effectiveness of antiperspirants:

There are many excellent deodorant bar and liquid soaps that have some antibacterial activity. Daily use of one of these products can cut down the bacterial counts in the underarm and groin areas. As discussed earlier, the only downside to deodorant soaps is that they tend to be harsher to your skin. If you develop irritation, you might try hydrocortisone 1% cream, which is an over-the-counter item that is safe and effective for mild dermatitis.

Absorbent powders are another way to fight body odor. Drying powders work by absorbing excess moisture and by placing a layer over the skin that helps prevent chafing. These are fairly effective at cutting down on excess free moisture but are not a good substitute for a real antiperspirant. If you wish to use one of these products, avoid those with corn starch since yeasts that cause candida skin infections live off the corn starch molecule.

If the strategies outlined above do not control your sweating body odor problem, there are a couple of additional measures you might try. Each of these may produce increased irritation, but you have to weigh the benefits against the side effects to determine whether it is worth it.

Aluminum chloride in high concentration. Antiperspirants containing aluminum chloride in higher concentrations are available by prescription. These agents control sweating very well, but almost no one would volunteer for the inflammation that usually ensues.

Iontophoresis. For reasons that are far from clear, if you run an electric current through the skin containing sweat glands, those glands can be turned off for days. There is a commercially available apparatus configured to fit under the arms. Two or three treatments per week, each lasting about 30 minutes, are usually sufficient to control even problem sweating. If this interests you, consult your dermatologist for more information. By the way, please don't jerry-rig one of these devices yourself. Electrocution is an effective but draconian way to treat increased sweating.

Shaving the underarms. For women, this is a simple alternate approach to the problem of underarm odor. Apocrine sweat and bacteria stick to the axillary hair, so removing it reduces the odor-causing elements. If you are a man, you have a harder choice to make. In our culture, underarm shaving is considered a feminine activity and being hirsute, including in the underarm area, is a part of the masculine persona. I have never conducted a scientific poll on the subject, but I suspect that once it was understood that hair in the axilla contributes to underarm odor, people would prefer to deal with a man with cleanly shaved underarms and no odor rather than a hairy man who smells like a locker room.

Sweaty and smelly feet are common and distressing; just ask a shoe salesman. In most instances, good foot hygiene is sufficient to control the problem. Here are some general guideline:

- Whenever possible, wear shoes of lightweight materials that breathe. Sneakers absorb moisture, but if you wear them for seventy-two hours straight they get a little foul, and so can your feet. Avoid shoes made of synthetic materials such as vinyl. These shoes keep a great shine, but the odor can get very strong.

- Rotate your shoes. Try to wear a given pair once every three or four days. It will give your shoes a chance to dry out.

- Wear cotton socks and avoid heavy wool socks. Going without socks may turn your shoe lining into a permanent repository of vile odors. You might try to spray the insides of your shoes with a fragrance that masks odors.

- Insoles with absorbent materials such as activated charcoal can absorb sweat and odors. These can be purchased at the foot care display in the supermarket.

- If your feet sweat too much, try using your antiperspirant on them, particularly in the toe web spaces; these are sites where sweat and bacteria can build up.

There are a few unfortunate individuals who have a severe sweat problem limited to the palms and soles. In some, this occurs only in times of stress. In others, it is a continual problem. Picture for a minute a person squishing in his shoes as he walks down the street or turning his palm down and producing droplets of sweat on command. This is not a pleasant way to go through life. If you have this degree of dysfunctional sweating, you need to see your dermatologist. She may recommend the iontophoresis apparatus described above or one of a number of strong chemicals to be applied to the palms and soles. Unlike the underarms, the skin of the hands and feet is relatively resistant to the inflammatory effects of harsh agents.

Desperate people often seek multiple opinions to solve difficult medical problems. I have a bit of advice for you. Avoid seeing a surgeon for your palm and sole sweating problem. There is a surgical procedure, cervical sympathectomy, which permanently removes the nerves that innervate the sweat gland of the palms. Although this sounds like an acceptable solution, the improvement is usually only temporary. Then you are stuck with an irreversible nerve loss.

If your sweat problem is terrible and is limited to the underarms, a surgical procedure can be performed to remove the bulk of the apocrine glands in those areas. This is an effective way to improve the situation, but the operation is costly and the result is that you may not be able to raise your arms over your head because of the scar tissue that forms after this kind of operation.

Hair Removal

Although styles and cultural norms are changing constantly, most of us have hair someplace on our bodies that we would prefer to hide or remove. We are all familiar with the various methods available. This section will outline our alternatives and discuss the most efficient means of accomplishing this end.

SHAVING

For most of us, this is one of life's little tasks that we do almost unconsciously and consider it a minor nuisance, at best. The cosmetic industry has provided us with many effective and fairly gentle tools so that the days of going to work with eighteen little pieces of toilet tissue covering razor nicks is largely a thing of the past. For those of you who are not satisfied with the quality of the shave that you are getting or are on the lookout for the "perfect shave," let us review some important tips for shaving.

Men have several types of razors to choose from. Those who prefer a traditional blade over an electric razor should opt for the new double-edge variety. A good blade can last for seven to fifteen shaves, depending on your beard type. However, replacing your blade after ten shaves is a good rule to follow.

For those of you who prefer an electric razor, which is gentler on men with skin problems in the beard area, there are three types of electric razors to choose from. The foil-head razor has a screen over the cutting head that moves back and forth as you apply pressure to your skin. The second type has spring-mounted guards over the blades, and the third is a hybrid between an electric and a blade-type razor. It has disposable double-edged blades and a battery-driven vibrating head, which moves the blade independently of what you do by pulling the razor across your face. All of these razors will give you a decent shave. If you like electric razors but are troubled by razor burn, try the hybrid product.

Some men have naturally curly beard hair that leads to ingrown hair and a condition known as pseudofolliculitis barbae (shaving bumps). Individual hairs curl back into the skin and produce foreign body reactions that can ultimately scar. For individuals with this problem, the cure is to grow a beard. If one lets the hair grow long enough it stops curling back into the skin. For those whose job or social situation prevents them from growing a beard, there are ways to minimize the ingrown hair situation. Chemical depilatories are fairly effective; however, many people cannot tolerate the irritation associated with their use, however. Specially designed razors and shaving gels are now available and are somewhat useful. If you use this approach, try to shave every day. This sounds contradictory to the notion that shaving causes irritation, but here is the rationale: If hair is allowed to grow, it will curl inward into the skin. If you shave every day, the beard hair never gets long enough to do this. If you do use blades and shaving cream, always shave with the grain. For those with an intractable problem, electrolysis is one solution. More about this later in the chapter.

There has been some recent interest in the use of alpha hydroxy acids for the management of pseudofolliculitis barbae. Daily applications of an 8% AHA cream or lotion supposedly helps flatten the shaving bumps and keep them from recurring. This is worth a try if you suffer from this malady.

Women have slightly different hair removal problems than do men. The hair-bearing areas tend to be less densely populated with hair follicles, but even a minimal amount of growth is often unsatisfactory. There are several different options, depending on your expectations, motivation, time to devote to the enterprise, pain threshold, and amount of disposable income.

Shaving is a reasonable alternative for women as well as men. First we need to dispel a myth that makes some women hesitant to use this technique: *Shaving the hair does not make the hair grow more rapidly.* Hair grows from deep in the skin and is totally unaffected by what happens at the surface. It is a similar situation to cutting the grass; you shorten the individual blades but do nothing to affect the growth rate. If you wish to shave daily, do it. A number of shaving products are targeted for women, including razors and shaving gels. As far as I can tell, the only substantial difference between male and female shaving products are the packaging and the color of the shaving instruments, the size of the handles on the razors, and the smell of the shaving creams. Don't feel less feminine if you can buy men's shaving products on sale for your own use.

Many women complain that when they switch from another method to shaving as a means of hair removal, the hair becomes coarser. What is happening is that the hair is being cut perpendicular to the skin, which creates a rough tip that feels coarse. Some women view shaving negatively because they have to do it so often to keep the skin feeling smooth. Since this technique does not cut hair below the surface, the hair emerges soon after shaving. If you prefer other methods to shaving for care of unwanted hair, you have several options.

BLEACHING

Bleaching is the simplest and least expensive of the alternatives for concealing unwanted hair. This works very well for fine hair, particularly on the upper lip, sides of the face, and forearms. Repeat bleaching works by damaging the hairs to point where they break off. Commercial products are available, but you can also prepare your own solution by mixing 6% hydrogen peroxide with ten to fifteen drops of ammonia. Apply immediately because the solution starts to lose its potency soon after the chemicals are mixed. If you have no irritation, leave the solution in place for thirty minutes before washing off with soap and water. If there is a burning sensation, wash it off promptly. There is no harm in bleaching the hair as frequently as you want. Watch for one possible pitfall of bleaching: your bleached hair may stand out when you tan.

CHEMICAL DEPILATORIES
Chemical depilatories effectively remove hair, even a little below the skin surface. These products are specially formulated for either the face or legs. There are differences, so you will need to use the products for specific use. These agents contain chemicals that split the chemical bonds and lead to breakage of the hair. They can produce skin irritation, particularly on underarm skin. If irritation is mild, you can relieve it with hydrocortisone 1% cream used after each depilation. The only other potential negative with these products is the unpleasant smell, which can be only partly masked by added fragrances.

Chemical depilatories come as lotions, creams, or powders. Application instructions vary, but most require that you leave the preparation in place for five or ten minutes, then remove with water. These work so efficiently that you may need to use them only every one to two weeks.

WAXING
Waxing has been used for centuries to remove unwanted hair. A thin coat of warm, liquefied wax is applied and allowed to cool and solidify. Hairs become embedded in the wax. When the wax layer is stripped, the hairs are yanked from their roots. The advantage of this form of depilitation is that it needs to be done less frequently than other methods because the hair is plucked from deeper below the skin surface. The disadvantage is that it can hurt like crazy to have your hairs ripped out. Another slight disadvantage is that the emerging hairs must reach at least a certain length before this technique can be employed. Thus, you will have to endure some stubble before using this technique.

Home waxing kits are available, but be prepared to hurt yourself. There is a correct way to do this to minimize the chances of adverse events, including burning the skin and painful inflammation of the hair follicles (folliculitis). Seriously consider letting a professional at a salon perform this service for you.

PLUCKING AND TWEEZING
Plucking and tweezing individual hairs is a reasonable, if somewhat painful, way to remove them. This will not cause the hairs to grow back

faster or coarser. Use of specially designed instruments is the preferred method. One such instrument is an electric tweezers that is essentially a sophisticated plucking device. It works, and might save you some time and effort.

There is a device on the market that plucks the hair mechanically with a rapidly rotating wire loop. Theoretically, this could be an efficient way of plucking many hairs quickly. However, there is a definite risk of severe skin irritation, particularly folliculitis, which makes this method dicey at best.

ELECTROLYSIS

The only permanent method of hair removal is electrolysis. The roots are destroyed by the heat generated by an electric current. This is done by inserting a fine needle attached to a thermolysis apparatus into the pore containing the unwanted hair and sending the current through the needle. About 50% of hairs treated this way will not regrow. However, the other 50% will need to be retreated, sometimes multiple times. The whole process is painful, costly and time-consuming. The success is also very operator-dependent. If you choose this method of hair removal, don't pick the name of an electrologist out of the phone book at random. Talk to others who have undergone the procedure to get their recommendations. Your family doctor may also know of skilled persons in this field.

There are problems associated with this technique, even in the best of hands:

- Damage to the surrounding tissue around the destroyed hairs can produce ugly scars or pigmentation.

- There is a chance of infection after electrolysis.

- It is technically more difficult to eradicate curly, wavy, or kinky hair because the follicle is curved; this makes it difficult to place the needle. If you have this type of hair, pick an electrologist with experience with your hair type.

- This is a slow and tedious process. It is best suited for small areas of excess hair such as the chin or upper lip. Life is too short to depilate your entire legs.

Home electrolysis devices are available for the person who would like to hurt herself while not removing many hairs in the process. First, the technique requires a great deal of skill. You may be dexterous, but unless you have a great deal of experience, it is highly unlikely that you will be successful. Second, the most popular tweezer-type devices don't get deep enough into the hair follicle to do enough damage to the hair root. Very few health care professionals would dream of doing this to themselves or suggest that their patients use these devices.

Nail Care

Our nails catch the brunt of the abuse that daily living doles out to our hands and toes. The hard nail protein protects the fragile fingertips and helps us grip objects. Nails are made of tough keratins but still need some routine care to stay in top shape. If you wish to keep your nails looking their best, consider these guidelines for routine maintenance:

- Minimize your hands' exposure to water. When you must expose your hands to water, try to wear protective cotton-lined rubber gloves. Water removes the protective coating from the nails and paradoxically causes them to dry out.

- Apply a moisturizing cream to your nails at least once daily. Products containing alpha hydroxy acids might give you a slight additional benefit.

- Wear gloves when doing chores that might injure your nails. This is particularly true in the winter when your nails may be drier and more brittle.

- Avoid using your nails as tools. For example, don't dial a rotary telephone with your nails; use a pencil instead.

- Do not dig roughly under the nails to remove dirt and debris. This can be removed gently and automatically in the process of shampooing your hair, as you scrub the scalp with your fingers.

- Avoid manipulating the nail cuticle because this may scrape away the protective cells on the nail surface.

- Routine trimming or clipping of dry, brittle nails can cause them to split in several directions. Take advantage of the softening that occurs after bathing or showering to clip the nails. Toenails may need to be soaked for thirty to sixty minutes in water to soften them sufficiently to trim them without damage.

- Don't bother to try to strengthen your nails with nutritional supplements. There is no scientific evidence that gelatin or anything else can make much of a difference. There is a recent report that the vitamin biotin taken in large quantities can improve nail hardness. This seems to be true in horses, but I have grave doubts about it in animals that don't crave oats.

Many people choose to have nails tended to by a professional manicurist. In chapter 7, we will discuss specific nail cosmetics, but there are a few other things that you should keep in mind when having your nails done:

- Of all the cosmetic procedures performed at a beauty salon, none has more potential for real harm than a manicure or pedicure. This is true because it is not unusual for an overzealous operator to draw a little blood. This is a set-up for transmission of serious blood-borne pathogens such as the hepatitis virus and HIV. There are no uniform laws about the sterilization of equipment between clients; the individual shops are on their own. Here is where you must be a vigilant consumer. Insist that any instruments be appropriately sterilized before being used on your nails. Cleansing is not sufficient protection against spreading of these deadly viruses.

- Cosmetologists are good at manicuring the nails, but many don't know the first thing about the relationship between internal metabolic activity and nail appearance. A colleague of mine with normal nails visited numerous salons and was given advice such as: "drink more water, you need vitamin A and E supplementation, and you need to stop drinking milk." Several tried to sell her products to apply to her nails to give them additional strength. The moral of the story is this: Don't listen to everything your manicurist has to say about the state of health of your nails.

- Ask that the manicurist manipulate the cuticles of the nails as little as possible. The nail matrix is the area from which the nail grows and this sits, in part, under the cuticle. Any injury to this site could lead to a malformed nail plate. In addition, even minor trauma could allow infections to gain a foothold under the fold.

- If your nails are manicured frequently, they are probably being buffed repeatedly. This does give the nail sheen, but it may also thin and weaken the nail plate. You might suggest to your manicurist that once monthly buffing may be enough, unless this is done very gingerly.

Few habits are more common and more distressing than nail biting. It would seem to be a simple habit to break, but about 10% of adults habitually bite their nails. Many don't care what their nails look like, but, for those who are embarrassed and discouraged by the tenacity of the habit and the appearance of their nails, there is some hope.

Why do so many people insist on biting their nails? This has been the subject of considerable research that has resulted in numerous theories. The simplest and probably most accurate explanation is that this is a habit, plain and simple. No underlying psychological imbalance links the nail biters of the world. If you have this habit, take heart, you are no different from those of us who cannot resist biting our lips, scratching our necks, or twirling the curls in our hair.

Of all the "cures" proposed for this problem, the most effective methods are aversion therapy and what is known as response competition. The idea behind aversion therapy is to make biting the nails an unpleasant experience, to the point where you loose the desire to do it. The simplest way to accomplish this is to apply a bitter substance on the areas that are chewed on. One popular candidate for this job is quinine, but I am certain that you can pick your own poison. It is critical that the material be in place always for at least several weeks.

For those of you who would prefer to feel more in control of your behavior, response competition is a good method to try. The idea here is to substitute a competing behavior each time you have the urge to bite your nails. For example, try clenching your hand for three minutes each time you get the urge to work over your nails. This is a painless way to break this nagging habit.

4

The Search for
a Safe Tan

I t is a beautiful Saturday morning; the air is warm, a light breeze is ruffling the leaves, and the sun is shining brightly overhead. This is the kind of day that you dreamed of during the long, cold winter. Just as you are ready to greet this wondrous new day, you hear your mother's voice telling you to stay out of the sun. I am here to inform you that life is too short to miss out on its simple pleasures. If time outdoors is your passion, go for it. What I will advise is that there are problems associated with *excess*, unprotected sun exposure. Your skin has only a finite reserve against the sun's harmful rays. The strategy is to run your life as a marathon; don't use up this reserve in your early years, only to lament your behavior as you get older and wiser. In this chapter I explain how your skin reacts to sunlight, discuss sun burning and tanning, and then tell a few horror stories about the dangers of chronic overexposure to the sun's rays.

Photobiology

Solar radiation (sunlight) is emitted from the sun as a continuous spectrum of wavelengths. These are arbitrarily divided into regions. Cosmic rays and x-rays are very short wavelengths, and infrared and radio waves are very long wavelengths. The shorter waves are more energetic than the longer wavelengths. Between these two extremes are the ultraviolet rays. These invisible waves represent only 2 to 3 % of the total radiation reaching the Earth, but they are the ones that are responsible for most of the skin problems caused by sunlight.

The ultraviolet light spectrum is subdivided into three overlapping groups, UVC, UVB, and UVA. UVC is energetic and can damage the skin; however, it is completely absorbed by the ozone layer above the Earth. It is crucial to maintain this layer or else the sun's UVC rays could cause great harm to those who are chronically exposed. UVB is the part of the sun's spectrum that causes sunburn and is an important determinant in skin cancer formation and sun-induced skin aging changes. UVA waves do not cause sunburn, but are important in skin aging and may also be a cofactor with UVB in skin cancer production.

UVB light intensity varies greatly, depending on the time of day and the season of the year. It is negligible early in the morning and in the late afternoon, and it is greatly diminished during the winter. UVB peaks during the midday, especially in the summer. UVA varies less than UVB throughout the year. It peaks in the early afternoon.

When your skin is exposed to ultraviolet light, three things may happen: 1)Your skin may turn red, 2) there may be immediate, but temporary darkening of the skin, and 3) there may be delayed darkening (tanning). The response varies with the wavelength and intensity of the sunlight and with your skin's natural tendencies. UVB light causes reddening (burning) and tanning; UVA light causes no burning under ordinary circumstances but does cause tanning.

The ability to burn and tan is an inherent property of your skin. It is like a fingerprint. There is nothing you can do to change the way your skin functions when it is exposed to sunlight. A grading scale from one to six has been developed to categorize individuals by their ability to resist burning and produce tanning after UVB exposure. Type one people always burn and never tan, type three people burn moderately and tan moderately and uniformly, and type six individuals never burn and always tan. Although there is a rough correlation with skin color, it does not necessarily mean that because you are very fair-skinned, you cannot be a type three or four. This is how your skin functions, not how it appears.

Sunburn and Suntan

When you sit out by the pool and bask in the warm sunlight, your skin is working overtime to respond to the strong energy that it is absorbing. The first noticeable response is a slight redness that begins shortly after the exposure begins. This fades within thirty minutes of the end of your time in the sun. The real sunburn begins two to six hours later. It peaks at twelve to sixteen hours and fades in two or three days.

As mentioned above, UVB light is the culprit. The warmth that you feel on your skin as you sunbathe is from infrared rays, which do not cause the burn that you develop later.

Most of us do not sit in the sun in order to get a nice burn; we want to tan ourselves. This is also a two-phase process. Within minutes of exposure, there is an immediate darkening of the exposed skin, particularly in those with type three to six skin. Like the immediate reddening response, this only lasts a short time. The real tan appears in about two days and may last for weeks or months after exposure. Both UVB and UVA stimulate the pigment cells to make melanin, the pigment that causes your skin to look darker.

Before World War II, tanned skin was not considered to be particularly attractive or healthy. Tanned people were often considered to be in a lower social class because their occupations required that they toil outdoors, often in manual labor. For a variety of reasons, in the past fifty years, a bronzed body has become synonymous with the leisure class, good looks, vigor, athleticism, and youth. Nothing that public health professionals have done to try to change these notions has shaken these beliefs. My teenage daughter has heard me ranting about the bad effects of sunlight since she was a baby. She is still grilling me for my secret method of getting a good tan. (There are no secret methods.)

By definition, a tan is your skin's attempt to protect itself from the effects of the sun. If you get a tan, you have damaged the skin in doing so. Sun damage is cumulative. A little sun today, some more next week, a few hours next month—your skin remembers all this. Years later, long after you have stopped sunbathing, you will visit the dermatologist and insist that you don't go in the sun anymore. All the sun-damaged spots that are visible come from the old days when you didn't know any better. Mark Twain's lament that youth is wasted on the young will resonate in your mind but will not help you at all. You will not be able to go back and undo the damaging effects of the sun. Be different. Try to be *pale* and beautiful.

If you are serious about protecting your skin from the sun, there are many excellent ways to accomplish this and still enjoy an outdoor lifestyle. I am appalled when I hear well-meaning anti-sun zealots preach that your skin should never see the light of day. You will never get fat if you eat a diet of broccoli and turnips, either, but when does the fun begin with this kind of life? Don't limit your existence because of what the sun might do to you. Instead, incorporate the following strategies in your daily program and enjoy yourself.

TIMING OF SUN EXPOSURE

As mentioned above, the intensity of the sun's rays varies during the day. If you are outdoors in the early morning you might be able to stay out without burning for hours, while only a thirty-minute exposure at midday will cause a painful sunburn. Try to arrange your schedule to take advantage of the beautiful morning or late afternoon. Clouds do not completely prevent harmful UVB rays from hitting the Earth, so don't change your schedule just because there is cloud cover. You can burn yourself just as badly on a cool and cloudy summer day as on a sunny and hot one. You may be tempted to get in a few extra holes on the golf course because of the moderate temperature, but, without protection, you can burn.

PROTECTIVE CLOTHING

A farmer who has practiced his craft for many years will have a sharp cutoff between the rough, scaly, thickened skin of his neck and the smooth, unblemished skin of his upper back. Decades of neck exposure to the sun have produced the damage there, and years of covering the area of the adjacent back skin have protected this area from the damaging rays. Sun damage to the skin of the legs is common among women golfers but is seldom seen in men who play golf. Part of the reason for this may be that men are in the trees looking for their errant golf balls more than women. Even more important is that women wear skirts and shorts on the golf course, while, in many places, golf etiquette or custom requires that men wear long pants. Clothing is a good protection against the sun, so if you keep your shirt on and your pants long, a fairly large part of your skin will be protected from the sun.

For the exceptionally compulsive sun-avoiders of the world, a new line of clothing made with sun-blocking fabrics is being marketed. These fabrics block out almost all the incipient ultraviolet light to give the wearer absolutely maximum protection. This approach carries sun protection to an extreme that is entirely unnecessary for all but those few with an extraordinary degree of sun sensitivity. I doubt whether the farmer that was described above ever resorted to these types of apparel. His regular clothing protected him quite adequately.

SUNSCREENS

The single most important advance in the last twenty-five years in the fight against sun-induced skin problems has been new and better sunscreens. Improvements in chemical formulations and vehicle design have resulted in a diverse group of cosmetically elegant and useful products.

There are two general types of sunscreens. The most popular type involves chemical absorbers of ultraviolet light. These include PABA and its derivatives, the benzophenones, the cinnamates, and the salicylates, all of which work by absorbing ultraviolet light so that it doesn't damage your skin. Most modern preparations have two or more active ingredients to enhance the product effectiveness. Pure PABA has almost disappeared from the market because of the adverse publicity associated with it (due to allergic reactions and staining clothing) and because better chemicals have been developed. Most sunscreens contain PABA esters. These work mainly in the UVB range and partly in the UVA range. Benzophenones such as oxybenzone are usually incorporated in sunscreens with one of the PABA esters. These chemicals have some UVB-blocking activity, and they also block fairly well in the UVA range. Cinnamates and salicylates are seldom placed in sunscreens as a single agent. They are usually present with one or two other agents to boost the overall effectiveness of the product.

Many of the newest sunscreen preparations are physical blockers. The industry likes to call these "chemical free," as if chemicals are harmful and these are much safer. That these physical blockers do not contain chemicals is not what makes them special; they block out the sun's rays over a wide spectrum, giving you protection against UVB, UVA, and even infrared radiation (if this matters). This type of agent has been available for decades; it is what lifeguards apply on their noses to protect themselves and makes them look like clowns because of the heavy white color. The cosmetic acceptability has improved dramatically since cosmetic chemists have developed agents with a decreased particle size of the titanium and zinc, which are the active ingredients. With some effort, you can rub in the cream until it disappears. These are heavier and greasier than most chemical sunscreens. If not vigorously massaged into the skin, they can leave a fine, white film. This is a good choice if you don't mind working a little harder at applying the agent.

The efficacy of sunscreens in preventing sunburn is quantified by a number called the sun protection factor (SPF). It is devised in the following way: If you normally burn after thirty minutes of sun exposure, but with the sunscreen, it takes you twice as long to get red, the SPF of that agent is 2. If the SPF is 15, you would have to expose your skin fifteen times longer than without the compound to get the same sunburn. Many sunscreens have an SPF of 15 or greater. By using one of these products properly, you should rarely if ever get a sunburn again.

There is some controversy about whether there is a diminishing return once the SPF gets much above 15. You can buy a sunscreen with an SPF of 50. If you normally burn after thirty minutes, you could stay outdoors twenty-five hours without burning. This sounds like overkill, but there is another consideration. Protection against sunburn, skin cancer, and skin aging may not parallel one another. Although it is not known for sure, it is possible that more potent sunscreens may provide you with additional protection from the chronic effects of the sun.

The critics of sunscreens claim that these products are harmful and should not be used. Their argument is that because a person does not burn with sunscreens in place they allow the person to stay outdoors longer and damage the skin to a greater extent. This issue is not yet settled, but, if sunscreens do block out the injurious rays, the extra time in the sun may not necessarily lead to the damage predicted by these naysayers. Until you hear proof otherwise, use sunscreens. They are a marvelous way for you to enjoy the outdoors and minimize skin injury from ultraviolet light.

I am often asked if there is a "best" sunscreen. The answer is that there is a best sunscreen for you, but it may differ from one that another person may choose. Here are a few general guidelines that will help you pick the product that suits your needs:

- Try to use a sunscreen with an SPF of at least 15. If you find a product that feels good on your skin and it happens to have a higher SPF, that is fine, but don't choose a product that you don't like to use just because of a sky-high SPF. If you go to a sunny climate on vacation and wish to have a tan to show for all the expense and hassle, an SPF 15 sunscreen may disappoint you. Try one with an SPF of 6 to 8. This compromise will prevent you from burning and will allow at least some tanning to occur.

- If you sweat profusely or will be in water, use a waterproof preparation. This is a big selling point of many products. You should have no difficulty identifying which products have this property. Prolonged immersion in water does decrease the protective power of even the waterproof brands. Reapply your sunscreen frequently if you go in and out of the water.

- Many people who wear wide-brimmed hats are under the false impression that these are as good as sunscreens. Ultraviolet light bounces off water, sand, snow, and pavement. Hats do not provide adequate protection in these situations. Even if you sport a giant sombrero, use a sunscreen.

- Over one half of the total sun exposure that you get occurs in the first decade of your life. It is critically important to insist that your children get in the habit of applying sunscreens just as they learn to brush their teeth daily. Remember that when your children are at school, they still go outside for physical education class and for recess. They need sunscreens every day. There are several sunscreen brands that are marketed specifically for children. However, there is nothing in "adult" sunscreens that can't be applied to children's skin. Make life less complicated for yourself. If your children like your sunscreen, let them use it.

- I often hear from apologetic patients that they would love to follow my advice and use sunscreens but they are allergic to *all* types. Sunscreens differ from one another in chemical composition and vehicle delivery system. Nobody is allergic to every conceivable combination of ingredients. There is a sunscreen that you can use safely and effectively. Ask your dermatologist to give you starter samples of different products. At least one of these will work for you.

- The only beneficial effect of sunlight is that it causes the synthesis of vitamin D in the skin. The argument has been made that heavy use of sunscreens could cause one to become deficient in vitamin D. It is virtually impossible to become vitamin D deficient if you have even a marginal diet. It is added to all dairy products. I have never come across a person who used sunscreens so thoroughly that none of his skin got any ultraviolet light, and at the same time had a diet that contained insufficient quantities of this nutrient. I doubt whether such a person has ever existed. If you are not convinced, take a multivitamin supplement containing vitamin D.

Tanning Aids

For those of you who wish to take a more active role in changing your skin color to a darker shade, several different approaches have emerged to help you along. These are referred to as "tanning aids," because they are supposed to give one's skin a tan color. In some instances, the color produced has only a passing resemblance to the one you get from sun exposure. A more appropriate description for these approaches might be "skin-coloring aids."

The safest way to achieve a tanlike color on your skin is to use one of the skin stains. They are colorless creams or liquids, usually containing dihydroxyacetone, that combine with the proteins on the top of the skin to produce a brownish hue. When applied evenly, the color can resemble a tan fairly well. If you do not apply these products neatly, your skin will have a streaky brown appearance. People may ask you if you were painting your house and got some of the paint on yourself. Even if you do not apply it smoothly, the skin color lasts only a few days, so there is no permanent damage done. The fact that the effects don't last is one of the problems with these preparations. Once you are on the program, you must keep using the product a few times a week to keep the effect. Repeated applications will cause gradual darkening, so you can customize the degree of darkening that you get. Don't aim for a deep brown color. The agents do not work nearly well enough to achieve this result. In the best of circumstances, your skin color will darken a few shades. If your goal in sunbathing is to darken your skin a moderate amount, you may find that these skin stains can give you a satisfactory result without the danger of sun exposure. However, unlike a natural tan, the tan from a bottle gives you absolutely no protection from future sun exposure. You can easily burn right through this stain.

Another way to stain your skin is to take a pill containing a colored agent that deposits in the subcutaneous tissue. The most popular of these is canthaxanthin, which is a carotenoid that is a distant cousin to vitamin A. Carotenoids are part of what gives carrots their orange-yellow color. If you would like to look something like a carrot, these products are just right for you. Only a color-blind person could fail to see that the "tan" has not occurred naturally. Besides the less-than-optimal hue, canthaxanthin has caused some adverse reactions that have led to its removal from the market in the United States. It is still available from mail order catalogs, but I would recommend that you find another way to express your individuality.

Tanning accelerators are another popular substitute for the sun. The main building block of melanin, the coloring pigment in our skin, is the amino acid tyrosine. Several years ago, some bright scientists figured that, if large amounts of this amino acid could be added to the skin, the pigmenting reaction would move more vigorously and a darker tan could be achieved. There is one major problem with this reasoning. The skin already has plenty of tyrosine, more than enough to make large amounts of melanin. The rate-limiting step in melanin synthesis is the conversion of tyrosine to the next step in the reaction by the enzyme tyrosinase. To increase pigmentation naturally, this step must be promoted.

Experience has shown that tyrosine-containing products do not increase tanning. They are useless products, and there is no reason to waste your money on them. If you don't believe me and wish to try them yourself, note that you still must get sun exposure for the supposed reaction to take place. You are not sparing your skin by using these tan accelerators.

Throughout this book, I have resisted the temptation to stand on a rhetorical soapbox and preach to the congregation. I must deviate from this policy this one time, because the issue of tanning salons is too important. Tanning booths are one of the most pernicious industries to make its way to our shopping centers and health clubs. They were introduced as a safe alternative to sun bathing for those who wanted a tan. There is one problem with this idea: *There is no such thing as a safe tan.* (If you want a safe alternative, try a skin stain.) Tanning booths have high-energy UVA bulbs that damage the deep layers of the skin. The big lie that tanning salon owners tell you is that UVA cannot cause skin cancer. That is not correct. UVA may be a major promoter of skin cancer. They also say that you should not worry about premature skin aging. Wrong again! UVA is the part of the sun's spectrum that does just that. The wrinkled and withered thirty-year-old people that I see as patients here in Arizona have UVA light from the sun to blame for their troubles. The tanning salon industry has now exported this problem all over the world. You now do not need to live in a sunny climate to ruin your skin early in life. Chronic exposure to tanning bed UVA light will do it for you, even in the winter.

Most states have poor regulatory authority over these devices. Many tanning salon owners haven't the faintest idea of exactly how much energy is coming from their bulbs. When you go into the booth, you may be getting gigantic doses of UVA. There is no way for you to know, since UVA does not cause burning.

If you or your children are looking for a public service to perform, one where countless people might be spared future health problems, try picketing your neighborhood tanning salon. Perhaps they will be forced to face the public scrutiny that they deserve as purveyors of a public health hazard.

Adverse Effects of Sun Exposure

Throughout this chapter, I have been alluding to the problems that the sun can cause your skin. These can be divided into those that occur after a single large dose of sunlight, and those that appear after chronic exposure over many years.

SUNBURN

All of us are familiar with the painful, red skin that we face after a day of fun in the sun. Most such burns are first degree; they have redness and swelling, but there is no blistering. Severe sunburns can produce second degree burns where there is blistering. Rarely, one can get a third degree burn from the sun where there is full-thickness destruction of the skin. These burns are not qualitatively different from one that you would get if you touched a match to your skin.

If you do develop a mild sunburn, here are a few simple things to do that will give you some relief:

- The treatment of choice for all burns is soaking in ice water, preferably done immediately after the burn has been detected. These can be applied for twenty minutes twice daily for the first day or two.

- Apply lubricants liberally twice daily. These will be soothing and will make the peeling phase a little less noticeable.

- Avoid burn remedies that contain anesthetics. Some people become allergic to these preparations, and they don't work that well anyway.

- Many people swear by aloe gel for minor burns. They are, at the least, cooling to the skin, and they might also speed healing somewhat.

- If you fall asleep under a sun lamp or at the beach and are sure that you are destined to sustain a serious burn, contact your doctor. He may suggest that you take corticosteroid pills for a few days to try to abrogate the inflammation in the skin before it establishes a foothold. This aggressive form of therapy is not indicated for most ordinary sunburns.

- If you develop a blistering sunburn, consult your doctor. There are several topical and systemic treatments that he may use to prevent infection and to promote uneventful healing.

PREMATURE SKIN AGING

Over the years, your skin deteriorates like the rest of the body. However, a great deal of what is interpreted as aging is really sun damage, which gives your skin the appearance of someone older. I have known many people with beautiful skin in their eighties and many others whose skin was ruined before age forty. Heredity plays some role in this, but chronic sun exposure is primarily the culprit.

There are several telltale signs that you can search for to determine how much the sun has aged your skin. None of these changes indicates a serious medical problem. They do indicate that you have received enough sun exposure to permanently change the skin's structure:

- A thick, leathery feel with exaggerated crosshatches on the surface. This is most commonly noted on the back of the neck and on the tops of the forearms. Compare the sun-exposed side of your forearms with the underside of these extremities. If there is a big difference in texture, you are sun damaged.

- Irregularly pigmented splotches on the sun exposed skin. These are solar lentigos (see chapter 5).

- Easy bruising after minor trauma. This occurs mostly on the forearms. It happens because ultraviolet rays degenerate the connective tissue that supports the skin's blood vessels.

- Irregular, yellow-white bumps that coalesce into plaques on the sides of the forehead and neck. This is called solar elastosis and occurs because of degeneration of the collagen fibers in the upper part of the dermis.

There are several things that you can do to minimize the problem you have. Since sun damage is cumulative, even if you have had much previous sun exposure, it is still worthwhile to change your habits to reflect a more healthy respect for the sun's capacity to injure the skin and make you look older. In chapter 8 I outline several alternatives for correcting some of this damage either with medications or with surgical procedures.

ACTINIC KERATOSIS

If you are a fair-skinned person and spend enough time in the sun, it is highly likely that you will develop one or more red, scaly spots on your face or upper extremities. These are actinic keratoses. They come as a result of sun damage to the cells in the epidermis. These lesions are theoretically precancerous; occasionally, they may degenerate into a type of skin cancer, squamous cell carcinoma. The likelihood that one of these lesions will turn into a skin cancer is not high, but if you have hundreds of these keratoses, as many people do, your odds increase dramatically. They also are a marker that you have been exposed to the sun for a long time and that the entire sun-exposed skin is at risk for skin cancer.

Actinic keratoses are not a worrisome condition. In fact, approximately 40% of these lesions will regress in about six months without any treatment. There are good reasons for treating some of these lesions, however. The two best indications are discomfort and rapid growth. Another reason to have these treated is the fear of skin cancer if they are allowed to remain. This last indication is not that strong, since the vast majority of actinic keratoses never change into skin cancer. Watchful waiting is an entirely appropriate approach to the problem of actinic keratosis.

If you wish to have these keratoses treated, there are several alternative methods to consider. Here are two popular ones:

- Cryotherapy is the application of a cold substance (liquid nitrogen) that causes the treated site to blister and to slough. With it goes the keratosis. This is a good method for individual spots. If you have numerous lesions, this method becomes somewhat impractical and is quite expensive, since your physician will probably charge you by the number of lesions treated. Cryotherapy often leaves small white scars. Since many actinic keratoses are located on the face, you have to decide if you are willing to risk this outcome to rid yourself of a benign growth.

- For those with numerous actinic keratoses, fluorouracil (5-FU) is a method to get rid of them without treating the lesions one at a time. Fluorouracil comes as a cream or lotion and is applied for three to six weeks. The drug selectively acts on the actinic keratoses and does not affect normal skin. If you have one hundred lesions, only those spots will react to the drug. The only problem with this approach is that the medication causes a great deal of irritation; that is how it works. You will definitely look worse before you look better. Your skin gets red, sore, and crusty and stays like that for a couple of weeks. You will probably curse the dermatologist who gave you the medication in the first place. One half of all the irate phone calls I have gotten in my professional career have been from patients who could not believe that I would give them a drug like fluorouracil that would do a thing like that to them. It is well worth it, however. After the treatment is stopped and the reaction subsides, your keratoses will have vanished and your skin will look better than it has in years. Before you jump at the chance at using this wonder drug, you need to set aside a few weeks when you don't care about your appearance. Don't schedule a course of 5-FU therapy before a high school reunion. You will draw many curious stares from your former classmates.

SKIN CANCER

An epidemic of skin cancer is occurring in many parts of the world, especially in the United States and Australia, two places with a lot of sunshine and many fair-skinned people. There are now about 750,000 new cases of skin cancer diagnosed each year. It is by far the most prevalent form of cancer. This high incidence is directly related to the increased amounts of sunlight that much of the population has gotten over the past fifty years. There is also a genetic component that plays a role. If your parents had skin cancer, you are at increased risk for a similar fate. That has a lot to do with the fact that you probably share the same skin coloring as they do, giving you the same predisposing factor as they had. However, even if you have a family history of skin cancer, you are not condemned to follow in their footsteps. If you protect your skin from the sun, it is unlikely that you will have this problem. This is a truly preventable form of cancer.

There are two major types of skin cancer: basal cell carcinoma (BCC) and squamous cell carcinoma (SCC). BCCs are three-to-five times more common and are a little less aggressive in their growth pattern than SCCs. SCCs often arise in pre-existent actinic keratoses while BCCs arise from apparently uninvolved skin. Neither of these tumors has much potential to spread from the skin to distant organs.

A typical skin cancer appears as a sore that won't heal. It may bleed spontaneously, and it is often sore to the touch. On examination, it is a pearly color and often has a central crust. It may be as small as the head of a pencil or as large as a fist.

The problem with these tumors is that local destruction can occur if they are allowed to grow to a large size. Because of this danger, these lesions should be removed, preferably while they are still small. There are several effective ways to eradicate these tumors.

Electrodesiccation and curettage (E and C). This method is commonly used by dermatologists because it is quick, easy to perform, and effective at eradicating the tumor. Most surgeons do not like it because of the round scar that it leaves. Choose this method if you want a minimum of fuss and if finances are important, because this is one of the cheapest methods of skin cancer removal.

After the lesion is anesthetized locally, a sharp instrument called a curette is used to scrape down to the base of the lesion. An experienced dermatologist will know by feel when all the tumor is gone. An electric needle is then applied to the surface of the wound to cauterize any bleeding points. This sequence of curetting and electrodesiccating is usually repeated two or three times in rapid succession. The whole procedure should take about ten minutes.

Cryotherapy. In those patients who are poor surgical candidates, some physicians will use aggressive cryotherapy to freeze the tumor away. After the site is anesthetized, the operator will apply a spray of liquid nitrogen for one to two minutes. After the area thaws, he will repeat the procedure. The advantage of this method is that there is little or no bleeding. The main disadvantages are the extreme postprocedure swelling and inflammation and the delayed healing; it may take three months for the wound to be completely healed. Pick this method only if all other options are closed to you because of a concurrent medical problem. The side effects associated with cryotherapy are too great to recommend it for routine removal of skin cancers.

Surgical excision. Most surgeons and many dermatologists prefer to remove skin cancers by an elliptical excision. After the skin is anesthetized, a football-shaped portion of skin with the cancer in the center is removed. The defect is closed with two layers of stitches. The main advantage of this method is that the resultant scar is a thin line. If the surgical excision is placed strategically in a skin fold or wrinkle, you may not be able to find the scar after several months. Another advantage is that the whole specimen can be evaluated by the pathologist to assure you that the entire cancer is gone.

Excisional surgery is more involved that either E and C or cryotherapy. The procedure may take up to an hour to perform. In addition, there must be a return visit to remove the stitches. This method is usually considerably more expensive than the others. If cost is not a consideration, and you want the least noticeable scar, this is the approach to use.

Radiation therapy. If you are a poor surgical candidate and have a lot of free time, radiation therapy is a good approach for you. Skin cancers are very radiation-sensitive, so most can be successfully eradicated this way.

Radiation is given in small increments over a couple of weeks. You may have to return for treatments ten or fifteen times over a three-week period. (Now you see why you need a lot of spare time to be able to complete this regimen.) The treatment has almost no side effects other than some discomfort as the tumor begins to melt away. The site usually heals with a mild scar. However, radiation scars always look worse with time. This is why this method is not recommended for those under the age of fifty.

Mohs micrographic surgery. For large tumors, or those that are regrowths after a prior procedure, there is a highly effective means of treatment. This is called Mohs micrographic surgery, named for Frederic Mohs, who popularized the technique many years ago. Only a few hundred physicians are trained in this technique. If you need this procedure, be sure to determine that your surgeon is a fully trained Mohs surgeon and is a member of the American College of Mohs Micrographic Surgery. There are many pretenders. If you are going to undergo this rigorous procedure, it should be from a practitioner who is skilled and experienced in it.

This technique involves the removal of small portions of tissue and examination of them under the microscope. With this method, all remnants of the cancer can be removed with almost complete assurance because of this microscopic control. Large amounts of healthy tissue do not need to be sacrificed to be certain that the tumor has been removed.

This is an excellent procedure for the tough skin cancers. It is not needed for most ordinary tumors. One might ask why not use this technique on every tumor since it is almost foolproof. The answer is that it is an expensive and time-consuming process. Skin cancer is not a serious enough problem to warrant the use of these resources, except in exceptional cases.

5

Common Skin Disorders

For those of you who are already feeling paranoid about today's health issues, here is a sobering thought: There are hundreds of maladies that affect the skin. Most are trivial and fleeting but occasionally serious or even life-threatening illnesses can occur. Aside from having its own set of problems, the skin can mirror illnesses that occur internally. A small bump on the skin could be a metastatic tumor from the lung, for example. In this chapter, I will discuss several of the most common skin disorders. I want you to know what these conditions are like and how to deal with them yourself. I will also show you what dermatologists have to offer in the way of therapy. In many instances, I will strongly encourage you to avoid professional assistance because either the condition is completely innocuous and self-healing or remedies that you can use on your own may be of equal benefit to what your physician may recommend.

I will say at the outset that I am a believer in the benefits of medical therapy for many skin disorders. However, the practice of medicine is an art. There are numerous ways to approach a problem. Social, economic, religious, and cultural circumstances often dictate the best approach for each individual. One person's skin reacts differently than another's. I am a scientist, but I still acknowledge that there are some miraculous and unexplainable things going on out there. What most might think of as a bizarre therapy may be perfect in your case. I no longer scoff at those who use bag balm, a treatment that farmers use for inflammation in cow udders. Too many patients have attested to its benefits in all sorts of skin disorders for me to ignore its potential as a therapeutic alternative.

There may be times when I give an opinion that is diametrically opposed to that of your trusted physician of twenty-five years. This does not mean that I am right and she is out of touch with reality. I have formulated my views based on what I have read and on my experience with patients. Your doctor may have a totally different opinion because her experience differs from mine. Please do not trot this book into your doctor's office just to show her how ignorant she is (or how ignorant I am) about the treatment of your skin problem. If a therapy that I scorn works for you, keep it up. You and your physician know what is best in your situation. My intention is to give you some alternatives. You should act on them depending on your individual needs.

The human organism has a remarkable ability to heal itself without our interference in the natural process. In addition, all therapies have some potential side effects associated with their use. I hope to persuade you to let nature run its course. Do not insist that your doctor treat you with something just to justify your trip to his office. I recently cared for a man who left disgusted with me for not giving him a medicine for a skin disease that he might get in the future. He viewed the visit as a waste of time because I didn't treat him with anything. I am not saying that you should avoid your doctor, but rather, in some circumstances, I will suggest that you give your body a chance to heal itself before scheduling a visit to your physician.

Acne

Acne is so ubiquitous that it is basically viewed as a normal part of growing up. At least 85% of all people will have acne at some time in their lives. Although this is considered a disease of teenagers, newborns can be afflicted to a mild degree, and women in their thirties are commonly bothered by it as well. For those of you who think you will never outgrow your acne problem, you can be assured that this is almost never seen after the age of fifty.

Acne occurs because of a dysfunction of specialized hair follicle, the sebaceous follicle. It is located on the face, chest, and upper back, the sites where acne occurs. As discussed in chapter 2, these follicles have giant oil glands and tiny hairs. The glands secrete an oily substance, called sebum, which is an important contributory factor in the development of an acne lesion. This material gets plugged in the duct of the follicle and results in whiteheads and blackheads. Blackheads are not caused by dirt. The color comes from the oxidation of the oils and from melanin pigment being released. Along with sebum, sebaceous follicles contain a bacterial species, *P. acnes*, which breaks down the oil to an irritating substance, free fatty acid. This breakdown product leaks outside the follicle and produces the inflammation that you see as a pimple.

This is a complicated disease with many different elements contributing to the predisposition to develop acne. There is a definite genetic tendency to have severe acne. As one of my associates once retorted to an irate patient who was frustrated that his son could not be cured: "I am a dermatologist, not a geneticist." Some people are destined to have a bigger problem than others. If one of your children has a severe acne problem, especially relatively early in life, your other children may be destined for the same fate. Acne seldom becomes a major problem before puberty because male hormones are central to the workings of the sebaceous follicle. Both boys and girls begin to manufacture androgens from the gonads at the time of puberty. These hormones stimulate the oil glands to produce copious amounts of sebum, which starts the chain of events that leads to acne. Women after menopause seldom have acne because this androgen stimulation is largely lost.

Medications taken for other purposes can greatly exacerbate acne. The most common offenders are lithium, used for manic depression; phenytoin (Dilantin), used in epilepsy; systemic corticosteroids, used for many diseases including arthritis and asthma; and iodides, present in some asthma remedies. People who never had major outbreaks previously may find that they have serious and uncontrollable problems when they are taking these medications. If your child is a bodybuilder and suddenly develops an uncontrollable eruption, consider the possibility that he is using anabolic steroids. These potent drugs increase muscle mass at the cost of severe acne, male pattern hair loss, and possible liver disorders. Certain oral contraceptive pills contain progestational agents that are relatively androgenic; these can also worsen acne. This is ironic since birth control pills are sometimes prescribed to improve acne. Therefore, it is important to know exactly what ingredients are in the medications that you take.

Certain environmental agents can make acne worse. Chloracne is caused by various chlorinated hydrocarbons. During the Vietnam War, soldiers who were sprayed with dioxin (Agent Orange) developed severe cystic acne; this product contained these hydrocarbons. Tar derivatives can also worsen acne. As noted in chapter 7, some cosmetics can produce a type of acne, aptly called *acne cosmetica*. Some people have flares of acne during hot and humid weather, a variant called tropical acne.

Hormonal derangements can result in recalcitrant acne. For

example, women who produce excess androgens in the ovary can have a severe acne problem. Clues to this diagnosis include abnormal menses, inability to conceive, and the onset of excess hair growth in a male pattern (hirsutism).

Teenage years are full of torment and angst as the child attempts to deal with the difficult business of maturing physically and emotionally. One consequence of this turmoil is a worsening of acne; this skin condition is definitely a psychosomatic disorder. This is another of the many examples that prove that life is not fair. A normal physical change in puberty produces acne, which freaks out the adolescent to the point where his emotional state makes the acne worse. Many children report that their acne improves in the summer. They think it is due to the beneficial effects of sunshine. In many of these young people, the release of the pressures of school may have more to do with the improvement than sunlight exposure.

There are several forms of acne but one lesion type is always present: the comedo. It is a collection of sebum, bacteria, and cells that forms a concretion in the duct of the sebaceous follicle. If the pore of the duct is widely dilated, it is an open comedo (blackhead, named because of the dark color). If the duct is not open, the lesion is flesh-colored and is called a closed comedo (whitehead). When comedos become inflamed, they become inflammatory papules. If there is pus inside the lesion, it is called a pustule. If the lesion is deep, red, and tender, it is an acne cyst. These are caused by a reaction to the sebum that has leaked out of the follicle. The person with acne often has excess facial oiliness, but this alone does not provoke the acne lesions. As I will explain, removing the oil does little to improve the acne.

There is no cure for acne; however, there are many effective ways to improve the signs and symptoms. The goal of treatment is to keep the acne down to a minimum until you outgrow (or outlive) it. One option for many people with mild flares is to postpone treatment. This is a reasonable alternative for the individual who does not care how his skin looks and prefers to avoid the hassles of putting medicines on his face for months or years at a time. My only problem with this approach is in the person with inflammatory lesions (red papules, pustules, or cysts). These can lead to scarring, even after a short bout of disease activity. A fourteen-year-old boy with skateboarding on his mind might not care about his skin, but it may matter a lot more when he is eighteen years old. It is for this reason that I try to persuade those with very inflamed skin to consider therapy. For the person with comedos only, there is no compelling medical reason to rush to therapy. I often see eleven-year-old children with three small pimples on their face, asking me to stop this process from becoming more serious. My approach is to ask the child if he wants to have the problem treated. If the answer is no, I will usually defer to his wishes. Early attention to mild acne does not prevent future major problems.There are many treatment choices for acne, so you must match the type and severity of the condition with the available options. If you have mild involvement with only a few pimples, consider skin cleansing and benzoyl peroxide before seeing a dermatologist.

A regular program of skin cleansing in those with mild acne will remove excess oils and will make the face feel better. Any of the mildly drying antibacterial soaps works well for this purpose. Acne is not a disease of dirtiness; you can't scrub it away. Don't spend half of your waking hours in the wash room with soap and water in hand. Washing the face twice daily is sufficient. Specially formulated acne soaps are not worth buying. For more on skin cleansing, see chapter 3.

The mainstay of acne therapy is benzoyl peroxide, a mild antibiotic available both by prescription and over the counter. It controls the bacteria in the sebaceous follicles. There is little reason to see a doctor just to obtain a prescription for one of these products since there is no meaningful difference in performance among any of these preparations. There are three concentrations of benzoyl peroxide (BPO): 2.5%, 5%, and 10%. The lowest concentration works just as well as the higher ones and is less irritating to the skin. There is no need to get different strengths for different parts of your skin or for more stubborn lesions.

BPO comes in various vehicles: gels, creams, lotions, and cleansing bars. Choose one of the gels or creams; avoid the BPO preparations in scrubs and cleansers. These are marketed for the person who gets irritation from the other agents. These scrubs are less of a skin irritant than the gels and creams only because they stay on your skin for only a short time. They do not work nearly as well as the products that remain in contact with the skin for many hours at a time.

BPO is a safe drug but does have some minor side effects. It can dry the skin and cause redness and flaking. Some interpret this as good news because they think the drug is working to dry out the acne. Removing the oiliness on the surface may make your skin feel better, but it does not improve the acne itself. Look at skin irritation as an adverse event rather than a therapeutic necessity. If a product causes chapping when applied twice daily, change brands or use your current one less frequently. BPO is a peroxide like the one in hair and clothing bleaches. If you get this on clothing, towels, or hair, it can bleach out the colors.

If, after six weeks of treatment with BPO and facial cleansing, you are not satisfied with your progress, it is time to consult a physician. The next tier of treatment involves prescription items and sometimes physical manipulation of the troublesome lesions. He will probably use one or more of the following approaches.

RETIN-A

If you have many comedos, Retin-A, or tretinoin, is the best treatment available. Its mechanism of action is different from that of any other medication. It breaks up the sebum plugs in the follicle and increases cell turnover. This causes the follicle to have a more normal pattern of keratinization. Retin-A is a synthetic vitamin A derivative, but vitamin A does not have any of the properties of tretinoin. Don't waste your time using topical vitamin A. It has absolutely no beneficial effects in treating acne.

Tretinoin is not an easy medication to use. Most people have at least some initial irritation with it. Your acne may worsen in the first few weeks of Retin-A use. The benefits take many weeks to become manifest. Using Retin-A takes patience and perseverance.

There are several strengths of tretinoin. In most cases, your doctor will start with a mild form and increase the potency after you become accustomed to the weaker variety. Retin-A comes in cream, gel, and liquid formulations. The cream is best for those with dry skin, and the gel is useful for people who have excess oil on their faces. The liquid is very drying and is seldom used.

If your doctor prescribes this medication, here are some general guidelines to observe:

- Apply the medication at night, at least fifteen minutes after washing your face. The irritant effects of Retin-A are more pronounced if the skin is damp when it is applied. Rub a tiny amount into the whole face, even those areas where there are no obvious blackheads or whiteheads. Avoid application near the corners of the eyes or the corners of the nose.

- If you are also using BPO, do not apply this in the evening because the peroxide will inactivate the tretinoin.

- Retin-A will make your skin more sensitive to the effects of the sun. This problem is somewhat minimized when you use the medicine only at night. There is still some residual effect the next day, however. It is important that you use a sunscreen if you plan to spend time outdoors. This does not mean that you should become a recluse for the months that you will be on Retin-A.

- There will likely be some chapping for the first two to three weeks. You can use a moisturizing lotion to minimize this problem. If this becomes too much of a bother, try the medication every other night for a few weeks, then revert to nightly use. The action of the drug is deep in your skin; peeling or chapping on the surface is not the goal of therapy. You should not have to endure this effect permanently.

- If there has been little improvement after about eight weeks, and if there has been minimal chapping, your doctor may increase the strength of the Retin-A.

- If it clears your skin completely, it must be continued to keep it looking good. You may be able to accomplish this with Retin-A use two or three times a week.

TOPICAL ANTIBIOTICS

For mild or moderate inflammatory acne, topical antibiotics are a safe and fairly effective choice. Don't expect miraculous results; be pleased if you improve by 50%. Several different drugs are used, including clindamycin, erythromycin, tetracycline, and meclocycline. None is substantially better than the others. Most physicians use erythromycin or clindamycin. Both come in several forms, including lotion, cream, and ointment. You can get them in roll-on bottles and in handy one-use pads. I would not recommend meclocycline because it has a strong odor. Tetracycline also has a peculiarity. It fluoresces when exposed to long-wave ultraviolet light, like the kind found in many night clubs. You could be unpleasantly surprised when your face lights up as the lights go on.

Benzamycin is a product that contains both erythromycin and benzoyl peroxide. It offers the convenience of a single application. The problem with this preparation is that it must be formulated by the pharmacist, which adds to the cost. It also must be refrigerated. Most people do not apply their acne treatments while in the kitchen, and it can be a nuisance having to go rooting in your refrigerator for your acne medicine late at night.

SYSTEMIC ANTIBIOTICS

If your acne is of moderate severity or beyond, you will probably need some systemic treatment. Nobody wants teenagers to take drugs for months or years on end, but sometimes it cannot be avoided. Acne lasts only a few years, but the scarring can last a lifetime. There are several options for long-term drugs.

These have been the mainstay of acne therapy for the past thirty years. They work by reducing the bacteria in the sebaceous follicles and reducing the inflammation in the skin. Since they only suppress the process and do not "cure" acne, patients can stay on them for years. The argument is made that chronic antibiotic therapy can cause those drugs to lose their effectiveness against other infections. This is true, but there are now so many excellent substitute antibiotics that the loss of one or two does not mean that a person will have inadequate defenses against future infections.

The most popular antibiotic used for acne is tetracycline. This is effective, safe, inexpensive, and easy for most people to use. The drug is usually administered twice daily until substantial clearing is achieved, then dose is slowly reduced. It takes four to six weeks to see real gains. What will be noticeable is that fewer new pimples will come to replace the old ones, which will slowly resolve. If you are given tetracycline, expect to remain on the drug for at least three months. If you do extremely well, your doctor may then stop this medication and substitute a topical antibiotic.

Although tetracycline has an impressive safety profile, there are still a few problems associated with its use. The medication must be taken on an empty stomach, which can cause stomach upset, particularly in the first few weeks of therapy. If this is a problem for you, try eating a cracker with each dose. Do not ingest dairy products within two hours of taking tetracycline. This will inactivate the drug. Women who are prone to vaginal yeast infections may find increased episodes while on this medication. The infections can be treated while you continue tetracycline, but if it becomes too much of a problem, another antibiotic is indicated.

Women on oral contraceptives are often advised that the use of tetracycline can diminish the effectiveness of birth control pills. I disagree with this notion and think that this is really only a theoretical possibility. However, if you cannot imagine becoming pregnant, another acne regimen is probably in your best interest.

There are rare instances of liver dysfunction in patients on tetracycline. For this reason, some physicians will order blood tests every few months. In my opinion, this is being far too careful. The chances of developing a serious liver abnormality on tetracycline are nearly zero. Perhaps if you promise not to sue your doctor if you develop a liver problem while on tetracycline, he might not order all those blood tests.

If you cannot tolerate tetracycline or if it does not work well enough, erythromycin is a good second choice. It is almost as effective as tetracycline, is fairly inexpensive, has few serious side effects, and can be used safely for years. The only common problem that people have with this drug is gastrointestinal discomfort, which can be temporarily disabling. It is initially taken twice daily, and the frequency can be adjusted downward as the skin improves. This drug gets absorbed better on an empty stomach. If it causes an upset stomach, it can be taken with food. Unlike tetracycline, dairy products do not inactivate erythromycin. This may be an important consideration in a growing child who drinks a lot of milk throughout the day and sneaks ice cream in the evening.

If two months of tetracycline or erythromycin fail to control the acne, there are more powerful antibiotics that can be used. Minocycline is a tetracycline derivative with increased fat solubility, which allows it to concentrate in the sebaceous follicle. It has the advantage of good absorption, even with food in the stomach. In addition, it does not make you sun sensitive. It is more expensive than tetracycline, although the cost has decreased since it has been marketed as a generic drug. Ask your doctor to write the prescription this way.

Minocycline is a safe drug but does have two side effects that can be troublesome. Some people complain of an upset stomach for the first few days of therapy, and, at high doses, many individuals develop headaches and dizziness. Fortunately, few people need the drug at this dose level. On rare occasions, it can discolor old acne scars a muddy gray, which may last for months after the medication is discontinued.

Clindamycin is another strong oral antibiotic that often works when weaker drugs fail. This would be used more frequently if it weren't for a rare but devastating side effect: diarrhea due to a bacterial toxin that appears in the large bowel. Although this happens in fewer than 1% of people who use this drug, its bad reputation has relegated it to the sidelines in most circumstances. This is an excellent antibiotic for acne. Since there is an effective treatment for the diarrhea when it is diagnosed early, I will treat patients with it if I trust that they will call at the first sign of trouble. In sixteen years, I have received exactly one phone call for this problem.

Other antibiotics are occasionally used for recalcitrant acne. These include trimethoprim-sulfamethoxazole (Septra, Bactrim), ampicillin, and various cephalosporins. Some people swear by these drugs, but there is scant evidence that they do much in most patients with severe acne.

HORMONES

In women with significant inflammatory acne, suppression of adrenal and ovarian androgens can turn around a potentially serious situation.

The estrogens in oral contraceptives and low-dose oral corticosteroids are used together to accomplish this end. This works best in those women who have increased circulating androgens, but it can be tried in others as well. This treatment is safe because of the low doses used; however, it is still a little daunting to be manipulating one's hormones to improve a skin condition.

ACCUTANE

If all else fails, there is still one last treatment left, and it is the most effective one that is available. Accutane, or isotretinoin, has changed the way acne is handled and has helped thousands of people whose acne could easily have ruined their lives. The drug is a synthetic derivative of vitamin A. It differs only slightly in structure from Retin-A but has greatly different characteristics. Isotretinoin dries up the oil glands and causes them to shrink. It also changes the way that the sebaceous follicle functions so that acne does not return even after the treatment is discontinued.

Accutane is indicated in those people with severe cystic acne that has not responded to at least one other systemic form of treatment. It can also be used in people without cysts but with new or impending scars from active disease. This is a potent drug, and the results of therapy are impressive. However, only a small portion of people with acne need it. In mild or moderate acne, its effects are not nearly as dramatic as in the more serious cases. Don't browbeat your doctor into prescribing this drug if she does not think it is right for you. Just because your sister benefited from this treatment does not automatically qualify you for a course of therapy. As you will see in the succeeding paragraphs, this is a hard drug to use. It has many side effects and needs close monitoring. Don't abuse it.

Accutane is given for four to five months. Longer treatment programs are of no added benefit, and shorter courses do not give one the maximum long-term benefit. One positive feature of Accutane is that when you start it, you can mark your calendar for the day the treatment will stop. This makes isotretinoin unique among acne therapies. At the end of the course, you will get at least a two-month drug holiday. The effects remain for months or longer, and often there is no further need for acne therapy.

Now that you are familiar with all the good features of this outstanding drug, it is time for the sobering news: Accutane has many side effects, some of which can be very troublesome:

- All patients have some degree of drying in the skin and mucous membranes. This doesn't sound like an important issue, but imagine having dry and extremely chapped lips for four months. Everyone on Accutane experiences this. If you wear contact lenses, you may have trouble because your eyes become dry and sore, and your contacts will add to the problem. Skin rashes can occur because of the dryness.

• About 15 % of those on Accutane develop sore muscles, most commonly in the low back and over the shoulders. This should not keep you from athletic pursuits, but you may need an occasional pain reliever to ease the discomfort.

• Some people on Accutane have mood swings. These are usually transient and mild, but I have treated one young man who became psychotically depressed while on this drug. His mind cleared within seven days of stopping the treatment.

• Occasionally, headaches occur, and they can sometimes be severe and unremitting. If this happens, your doctor will check you for a rare and serious side effect, increased pressure on the brain (benign intracranial hypertension).

• While on Accutane, your blood will be tested at least twice to determine if your cholesterol and triglyceride levels have risen. Since this is only a four- to five-month course of treatment, elevations of these fats in your blood are of little consequence. The only exception is the rare individual whose triglyceride level increases dramatically. This places that person at risk for inflammation of the pancreas (pancreatitis) and is an indication to stop the medication immediately.

• Isotretinoin can cause devastating birth defects in babies born to mothers who take it during pregnancy. Men who take Accutane are at no risk of causing birth defects in their future children. Women who take Accutane and subsequently become pregnant are at no risk once the drug is out of their system (about one month after the end of the course of therapy). As a precaution, *all* women of childbearing potential are given oral contraceptives or some other equally effective method of birth control before this drug is administered. Even those who are not sexually active need to observe this precaution. I have placed the daughters of two close friends on oral contraceptives. Both were thirteen years old at the time. Awkward conversations preceded the decisions to give these young girls a potent contraceptive drug, but it was absolutely necessary for them to be protected. Please don't quarrel with your dermatologist about this. The Food and Drug Administration requires this precaution.

OTHER ACNE TREATMENTS

Many other treatments are used for acne. Most are of historical interest only, because new therapies have superseded them. Others hang on because of the mythology associated with this condition.

Acne surgery. Your dermatologist may steal one of your prerogatives as a person with acne and pop your pimples for you. This is known as acne surgery. For those with many comedos, incision and drainage of many at a time can improve their appearance. It is debatable whether this has any long-lasting effect on the course of the acne. If you have inflamed cysts, your dermatologist may inject a low concentration of a corticosteroid directly into them. This will cool off the lesions and may minimize the scars. The injected material may cause a temporary dimpling (atrophy) at the injection site. Some physicians prefer the application of a cold substance, either carbon dioxide slush or liquid nitrogen, which causes superficial peeling and drying. Since acne is a deep dermal process, very little is accomplished by these techniques.

Ultraviolet light. When ultraviolet light is applied to the skin, it produces an inflammatory response that results in desquamation, or peeling. No peeling takes place in the sebaceous follicles where it is needed, so don't bother with this form of therapy.

Peeling agents. Many old-fashioned acne preparations contain drugs that cause superficial peeling. These include sulfur, resorcinol, and salicylic acid. Since Retin-A works so well, these agents are seldom used anymore. Some over-the-counter remedies still have these as the main active ingredient. Buy benzoyl peroxide instead.

Change of sexual habits. One myth that refuses to die is that one's sexual behavior affects acne in some way or another. Male sex hormones are important in the pathogenesis of this condition. However, increased sexual activity, including masturbation, does nothing to alter the amount of androgens that reach the sebaceous follicles.

Diet. The granddaddy of all myths about acne is that what you eat somehow affects your skin. The exact origin of this misperception is not known, but I have a theory. All kids eat junk food, including chocolate, french fries, and other forbidden edibles, and all kids have acne; therefore, junk food causes acne. A corollary to this thesis is that getting on a child's case for his bad acne that's caused by what he eats is one of the last remaining guilt trips that parents can lay on their offspring. This will set the matter straight. If a person is fed a high fat diet, he may gain weight but the oil content in his face will remain unchanged. Teenagers already feel bad enough about their complexions, and tying their behavior to this normal fact of adolescent life is not fair to them.

Eczema

One of the most common reaction patterns in the skin is superficial inflammation. The terms eczema and dermatitis are used interchangeably to describe these skin changes. When someone tells you that you have eczema, he is not giving a diagnosis. He is simply describing what he sees. An adjective must be added to categorize what type of dermatitis you have. It is important because the treatment may vary depending on the cause of the skin inflammation. In the succeeding paragraphs I describe what eczema looks like and discuss a few of the most common causes of this cutaneous reaction.

The earliest and mildest changes in eczematous skin are redness and mild swelling (edema). There is usually itchiness (pruritus) and occasionally a burning sensation. As the process progresses, there may be weeping and oozing. Scaliness, cracking, and fissuring often follow. If the skin remains inflamed for a long time and is so itchy that you rub it to an extreme degree, it may thicken and appear almost like tree bark. This is called lichenification and is one of the important hallmarks of this skin problem.

Two cutaneous diseases account for the vast majority of all cases of dermatitis; these are atopic dermatitis and contact dermatitis. About 15% of the population will be troubled by atopic dermatitis at some time. Another name for this entity is infantile eczema because it commonly occurs in the first few years of life. This is a genetic disease, but the pattern of inheritance is complicated. A tendency to develop one or more of a group of diseases is inherited. You may manifest atopic dermatitis, and your brother may have allergies or asthma. You may have a very mild disease lasting only a few years, and your children may have a severe, lifelong siege of eczema.

Although you may have allergies as well as atopic eczema, the skin eruption is not a manifestation of an allergic state. Consider atopic skin as being more sensitive to mild irritants rather than allergic to anything specific. If an atopic person wears a wool sweater, it will cause her incredible itching; if her skin dries out from too-frequent bathing, it will itch out of proportion to the degree of water loss. Some physicians believe that food allergies are responsible for the symptoms of atopic dermatitis. Elaborate food elimination diets are undertaken to try to pinpoint the culprits. With the exception of a few newborn infants who might benefit from a hypoallergenic diet, this approach is bound to fail. This is not an allergic disease!

The diagnosis of atopic eczema can be difficult. It can be confused with other eczematous diseases and certain infections. Unless you are absolutely certain of the diagnosis yourself, a consultation with a dermatologist could save you a great deal of unnecessary treatment of skin conditions that you do not have. As you will see below, once a program is outlined, you can care for yourself very nicely.

A typical child with atopic eczema first develops a rash sometime between six and eighteen months of age. The first sign that the child may be atopic is that his cheeks look very rosy. Initially, this is taken as a sign of robust health, but it eventually becomes clear that the redness is due to rubbing his face on his pillow and rubbing his itchy cheeks with his hands. From the face the pruritus and eruption spread to the neck and extremities. As the child gets older, the eruption may settle onto the hands and feet. Most people grow out of atopic dermatitis by puberty; however, many have this malady throughout their lives. In some people, atopic dermatitis flares in late adulthood. Many of these individuals had this problem in childhood, and this is a new outbreak of the same condition. Think of it as the start of a second childhood.

There is no cure for atopic dermatitis. The goal of management is to make you as comfortable as possible until your body is ready to rid itself of the condition. There are many effective ways to treat this problem. Treatment regimens should be tailored to fit your needs. What I outline here includes all the possible scenarios. Many will be helpful, but some won't be appropriate for you. Check with your doctor.

TOPICAL CORTICOSTEROIDS

The mainstay of therapy for all forms of eczema, including atopic dermatitis, is corticosteroid creams and ointments. When cortisone or one of its derivatives is given systematically, there are many serious side effects, but when they are administered topically, they are much safer. If you have mild atopic dermatitis, hydrocortisone 1% cream works well. It is inexpensive and can be obtained over the counter. If you have moderate or severe disease, this will not be strong enough for you.

For many people, prescription-strength corticosteroids are needed to control the disease. The most widely used product is a generic preparation called triamcinolone. It works much better than hydrocortisone and is also quite safe, even if used for prolonged periods. The exception to this rule is if it used on the face, where side effects can occur if it is applied for more than two weeks at a time. There are many brand-name competitors of the same efficacy class as triamcinolone. There is no reason to use these. They are not any stronger and will cost you a lot more money. For example, a sixty-gram tube of triamcinolone costs about ten dollars. The same quantity of a brand-name product may sell for thirty to fifty dollars. Pocket the difference and spend it on something useful.

If triamcinolone does not provide relief, there are stronger corticosteroid preparations. The effects are greater, but the risks of overuse are somewhat greater also. If you apply large amounts of these stronger drugs to involved skin for months, they could suppress your adrenal glands or produce some skin thinning. These things seldom happen, but you should be aware of the potential. Again, the generic agent, fluocinonide, will save you lots of money. Do not be afraid to request this from your doctor if he writes a prescription for a more costly alternative.

If you fail to respond to fluocinonide, there is one group of corticosteroids that is more potent. These so-called superpotent corticosteroids work better, but there is a substantial risk of side effects if more than fifty grams per week are applied to your skin. If you must treat 25% of your skin surface area, you will need far more than fifty grams per week. Most dermatologists avoid using these drugs in atopic dermatitis because the safety profile is not acceptable.

SYSTEMIC CORTICOSTEROIDS

In the person who does not do well on topical corticosteroids, these drugs can be administered by injection or in pill form, a much more effective way to treat the skin condition. You will likely remain clear while taking these medications; however, the risks are substantial. The following is a partial list of the potential adverse reactions that could ensue if you take an oral cortisone derivative such as prednisone for over thirty days: high blood pressure, increased susceptibility to infections, bleeding stomach ulcers, softening of the bones, diabetes mellitus, easy bruising, bad acne, cataracts, and muscle wasting. It is for these reasons that systemic corticosteroids should be reserved for only occasional use in recalcitrant eczema. It is tempting to go in for a shot once a month or to take a few pills daily to keep the skin problem at bay. You avoid having to smear all the messy medicines over your body; life is easier. There is a price to be paid for this approach. Your general well-being can be seriously jeopardized if systemic corticosteroids are overused.

ANTI-ITCH MEDICATIONS

Atopic dermatitis is one of the itchiest skin conditions known. The corticosteroids described above can relieve the itch to a great extent. Sometimes this is not sufficient, however. Many physicians recommend antihistamines for this purpose. These drugs do stop the itch of allergies where histamine, an irritating chemical in the skin, is the main culprit. But atopic dermatitis is not a histamine-mediated disease, so these drugs have limited usefulness. The main benefit of these medications is that they will help you to sleep through the night. In fact, antihistamines are the main ingredient in many sleep aides. If you are so itchy that it interferes with sleep, antihistamines are helpful. Diphenhydramine is a nonprescription antihistamine that serves this purpose well. Be careful if you use this during the day; it can really make you drag. There is no rationale for using the nonsedating antihistamines that are made for allergy sufferers. They do not reduce the itch of atopic dermatitis.

Many topical preparations claim to reduce pruritus. Most contain a counterirritant such as menthol, camphor, or phenol, which cools the skin. These are of marginal benefit in severe eczema but might help in mild cases. Avoid topical antihistamines. They don't work, and you might develop an allergic reaction to one of the ingredients.

OTHER TREATMENTS

Anything that is mildly irritating to the atopic person's skin will cause her to itch. Dry skin is the most common precipitating event for these people. Assiduous use of lubricating lotions and nondrying soaps and cleansers is helpful. For a complete discussion, see chapter 3.

Clothing styles change, but atopic conditions continue unabated. Stick with loose-fitting cotton garments. Even if designers dictate wool clothing, avoid it if you are atopic, because wool is very rough on atopic skin. Also, sweating can set off a paroxysm of itching. Wear as few layers of clothing as possible and avoid overheating.

Atopic dermatitis is a psychosomatic disorder. Your state of mind will often determine how severely you are affected. Many students flare terribly during final exams and miraculously improve during summer vacation. It is a hectic, tense world. Sometimes your body can signal to you when your tension level is creeping over the top. Listen to your body. If your atopic dermatitis suddenly starts acting up, consider your lifestyle and try to decelerate for a few weeks. Take a vacation, play with your dog, play with your kids, come home early from work, quit work (just kidding).

CONTACT DERMATITIS

Contact dermatitis is a skin inflammation caused by substances that come in direct contact with the skin. If you have eczema on your hands and feet, a product that you handle cannot be the cause of the problem since your feet never touch that material. There are two types of contact dermatitis: allergic contact dermatitis and irritant contact dermatitis. (For additional discussion of these two varieties, see Chapter 7.) Both will give you the same eruption. In allergic contact dermatitis, you develop an immune reaction to the material. Each time your skin touches this substance, even for a short time, it will react. In the more common irritant contact dermatitis, anyone could develop a rash if enough of the material were left on their skin for a prolonged period. These are materials like solvents, greases, tar derivatives, caustic substances, and acids. Here are some general guidelines in determining the origin of your dermatitis:

- Many people relate what happens in their environment to what they see on their skin. This is especially true with suspected cutaneous allergens and irritants. The most abused product that I hear about in my practice is laundry detergent. Countless people have blamed a change in their detergent for whatever they see on their skin. I suppose that there have been cases of contact dermatitis from these products, but they are rare. Many of these people have atopic dermatitis or dry skin. Since the reaction pattern is similar, it is easy to mistake contact dermatitis for other causes of skin eruptions.

- An accurate determination of the source of irritant or allergic contact dermatitis depends on good detective work on your part. If you suddenly break out on a Saturday, try to figure out what you handled on Thursday or Friday. It takes a day or two after the contact for the rash to appear. If you handled something new at 2:00 p.m. and broke out at 4:00 p.m., don't blame the new substance.

- If the eruption is in the shape of something that you have touched, this is a helpful clue. For example, if the rash is in the shape of your shoe strap, it is likely that a constituent of that strap is the culprit. The converse of this reasoning is, if you apply a preparation all over your skin and only break out in a small area, it is unlikely that a skin allergy is the cause.

- Skin allergies do not come and go. If you break out only 50% of the time after touching a substance, it is probably not the cause of your problem.

- Allergies to ingested foods are not responsible for allergic contact dermatitis. A common misconception is that "acid foods" or other food groups cause skin rashes. Certain foods can produce skin irritation or even an allergy when handled directly. This is an occupational hazard of chefs but not of diners.

Once you have determined the materials that are irritants or allergens, there are several things you can do before you seek professional medical attention. The first is to avoid the troublesome substance. This sounds like a kindergarten concept, but it is often not an easy task. This is particularly true of allergens that are present in all sorts of products. For example, chromates are a common constituent of cement, inks, matches, paper, and many other products. It is almost impossible to eliminate all contact with this ubiquitous substance. Many dermatologists can do allergic patch testing for suspected allergens. If the patches indicate that you have specific allergies, he will give you a list of common products containing these allergens.

For irritant hand dermatitis, decrease exposure to household irritants such as harsh soaps, bleaches, and solvents. When you prepare moist food, wear protective gloves. Lubricate your skin frequently to replace the protective oil layer that irritants remove. Several products market themselves as barrier creams. These supposedly put up a protective barrier between your skin and the environment, but they do not work as advertised. Some irritants are attracted to the barrier cream, which is exactly what you don't want.

Contact dermatitis is treated like atopic dermatitis. Topical corticosteroids usually are sufficient to calm the inflammation. If you have a dermatitis limited to the hands, you can maximize the effect of the corticosteroid by wearing wet cotton garden gloves for thirty minutes after each application of the cream. This hydrates the skin and allows the medication to penetrate better.

Moles and Melanoma

One of the ubiquitous spots on the skin of all people of all races is a pigmented spot, called a nevus (mole). This is a collection of pigment-producing cells (melanocytes) that cluster in nests. The average white person has twenty-five to forty moles; blacks have fewer such lesions. About 1% of newborns have one or more of these lesions. Most arise in the first two decades of life. They enlarge as the person gets bigger, then stabilize and remain unchanged until they begin to regress after age sixty-five. Nevi often darken during pregnancy and then revert to their natural color after delivery.

A typical nevus is a smooth, regular, uniformly tan-to-brown papule. It is usually less than 0.5 cm in diameter. Moles are most common on the sun-exposed surfaces above the waist but may occur anywhere.

Not all moles are small and uniform. Approximately 5% of white people have one or more atypical moles (dysplastic nevi). These are larger than 0.5 cm, have some color speckling, and have edges that are not sharply demarcated from the surrounding skin. They are composed of the same kind of cells that make up a normal nevus, but the configuration of the cells is slightly different.

Moles are benign growths. If they remain the way they start, they pose no risk to you. There is no medical reason to remove moles. They do not affect your health in any way. The only time that removal is suggested is when a nevus gets irritated by clothing and such. If you wish to have one or more of these growths taken off, it should be for aesthetic reasons only. Don't worry about your moles.

The situation with atypical moles is not quite as clear. These lesions are associated with an increased risk of melanoma in some predisposed individuals. Occasionally, the atypical mole itself changes into a melanoma. Does this mean that all atypical moles should be removed? Most would argue against this proposal because it would result in a great number of nevi being removed on the basis of a theoretical risk. I recommend to my patients that the worrisome moles be evaluated once or twice a year. If there are any changes that make me suspect melanoma, the lesion is biopsied immediately. If you choose to have a mole removed, there are two different approaches to consider.

Most dermatologists prefer shave removal because it is quick and simple. The spot is anesthetized with a local anesthetic such as lidocaine. The mole is then shaved off just below the level of the skin. No stitches are needed to close the wound, which heals from below after a few weeks. One pitfall of this procedure is that the scar is round and often depressed. It looks like a large chicken pox scar. The second problem is that the nevus can recur in cases where there are some deep cells that don't get shaved off. This results in brown speckling in the scar, which can be mistaken for a melanoma.

Some dermatologists and most plastic surgeons prefer to remove moles with an elliptical excision. After the site is anesthetized with lidocaine, a football-shaped incision is made in the skin around the mole. The incision goes down to the level of the subcutaneous fat, ensuring that all the nevus cells are removed. After the block of tissue is excised, the wound is closed with two layers of sutures. The resulting scar is a straight line. One advantage of this method is that the whole lesion is removed. There is essentially no chance that it will recur. The other benefit of this method is that a line scar is easier to cover than the round one that is the result of a shave removal. The disadvantage of this procedure is that it is more complicated and takes a more time to perform. It is more costly and requires a second visit to the doctor for suture removal. If you are not concerned about the appearance of the scar, opt for the shave removal. If the lesion is on your face and the scar can be hidden in one of your natural skin folds, an elliptical excision will ultimately look better.

Two other methods are sometimes employed in the removal of moles. One is burning off the lesion with an electric needle (electrodesiccation). This is a poor way to treat nevi for two reasons. A biopsy specimen is not preserved to corroborate one's clinical impression, and the scar is irregular and discolored. Don't allow this treatment to be used on you to remove your moles. The other method that is occasionally employed is cryotherapy with liquid nitrogen. This is an equally unsatisfactory way to treat moles because no specimen is taken for histologic examination and because the scar is often much whiter than the surrounding skin. Someone may try to sell you on this method because many moles can be treated in a short time. Resist the temptation to get rid of your nevi by this means.

One type of pigmented lesion that deserves attention is melanoma. This is a serious and potentially deadly form of skin cancer. This type of tumor arises from malignant melanocytes and can spread to distant organs. That's the bad news; the good news is that if caught in its early stages, melanoma is curable. These tumors are usually relatively slow growing; so you have some time to recognize the lesion and have it removed. This is one place where you can be a hero. I have cared for many patients with melanoma who are alive today because a spouse noticed a funny-looking black spot on their skin and insisted that it be examined. No one is expecting you to be an expert in sorting out what is a melanoma and what is a benign mole. Your job is to be suspicious of any spot that you think does not belong there. Here are some warning signals to help you decide what needs further attention:

- A previously stable mole that suddenly changes.

- A mole that bleeds spontaneously.

- A pigmented lesion that develops red, white, and blue hues (flag sign).

- A lesion that has an irregular shape or feathered margins.

- A mole that grows larger than 1 cm (about 1/3 inch) in diameter.

- A pigmented papule with a raised and flat portion in the same lesion.

Figure 5.1 is the only photograph of a skin lesion in this book. It has been included so that you can study it for comparison with skin spots that you or your family members may have. If you suspect that a skin spot is a melanoma, see a physician as quickly as possible. If you are going away for the weekend, don't change your plans. If you are planning on being out of town for a few weeks or more, don't postpone this office visit. It could save your life.

If your physician shares your suspicion, he will perform a diagnostic biopsy. If technically feasible, this biopsy will include the entire lesion. If it is too large, he may sample the most worrisome portion of the growth. If the pathologist who interprets the biopsy specimen under the microscope diagnoses a melanoma, your doctor will arrange to have the melanoma excised with a margin of normal tissue around it. If the whole lesion was removed for the biopsy, he will still recommend a re-excision to be certain that the whole growth has been removed.

After examination of the biopsy specimen, your doctor will be able to make some predictions about your prognosis. Thin tumors seldom cause problems, but thick melanomas are often fatal. The thickness of the lesion is the key to determining how well you will fare. Ask for the exact thickness of the tumor in millimeters. (A thin melanoma is one less than 1.0 millimeter thick; a thick tumor is one greater than 3.65 millimeters thick.) Keep that as a part of your personal record. If you should consult another physician about your tumor, she will want to have this information.

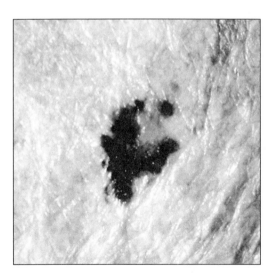

Figure 5.1   Melanoma of the skin. Note the dark color, irregular shape, and feathered margins.

Fungal Infections

The skin is a host to many organisms, including fungi. These usually live silently and undisturbed as colonizers. They cause no signs or symptoms of disease and are of no consequence. Some strains, however, are not content to live peaceably with the host. These are the pathogenic fungi, the source of the dreaded but fairly innocuous ringworm. This infection got a bad reputation many years ago when epidemics of fungal infections would sweep through classrooms and workplaces. With improved hygiene and living conditions, large clusters of cases are seldom seen, but it still remains a medical problem for many people.

There are three major types of organisms that cause skin disease in humans: candida, dermatophytes, and pityrosporum organisms. Each of these fungi has unique characteristics, and all are managed somewhat differently.

CANDIDIASIS

Candida organisms are the cause of what are called yeast infections. These usually occur in warm, moist areas such as the vagina, the mouth, and body folds such as under the breasts or in the groin. There is frequently a predisposition to develop this infection. Women who use oral contraceptives are at increased risk, as are those on chronic antibiotic therapy. Obesity is another risk factor since skin folds are a good breeding ground for the candida organism.

Infected skin is beefy red and often has small pustules around the margin. In men, the scrotum is a frequent site of involvement. This is in contrast to dermatophyte infections (ringworm) with which the scrotum is almost never involved. When a woman develops a vaginal yeast infection, there is a cheesy white discharge. If the mouth is infected, there are white patches, or plaques, that bleed when removed.

For minor candida infections, over-the-counter antifungal creams are very effective. A two- to three-week course of treatment is curative. In severe or recurring cases, your doctor may suggest that you take a systemic antifungal therapy. Attention must also be paid to the site of the infection. If the infected skin is constantly moist from sweat and so forth, drying powders can prevent relapses of the yeast infection. Be sure to avoid powders containing corn starch; candida organisms live off this material.

DERMATOPHYTE INFECTIONS

Humans acquire these common infections from the soil, from animals, and from other people. Not everyone who encounters the fungus will develop a full-blown infection. About 15% of the population lacks the immune defenses to ward off these organisms. These are the people who are bothered by chronic infections for months or years.

Dermatophyte infections may occur in the scalp, on the body, or in the nails. Mucous membranes are never infected. In the scalp, the lesions appear as partially bald areas with scale. Certain organisms can provoke a brisk inflammatory response; in these situations, redness and pustules will appear as well. On the body, the lesions appear as red, scaly plaques with an advancing red edge and central clearing, hence the nickname "ringworm." If the nails are affected, there is scale underneath the nail plate, and the plate itself is often discolored and misshapen.

Localized infections of the body can usually be treated with one of the antifungal creams purchased without a prescription. These include those containing clotrimazole or miconazole. Other agents are available by prescription, but for the most part, they are not significantly better than those you can buy over the counter. If these do not work well, consult your physician. You may not have a fungal infection after all. One of the most common diagnostic errors I see is calling something a ringworm infection. There are many other skin diseases that have a red, scaly appearance. When in doubt, do not treat for fungus; you will be wasting time and money.

If you have a scalp infection, systemic therapy is necessary. There are several prescription drugs that can clear the infection in six to eight weeks. The most widely used medicine is griseofulvin. This is safe and fairly effective in most scalp ringworm infections. A course of treatment may cost you over one hundred dollars, which is a lot to eradicate a minor fungus. Unfortunately, topical therapy does not work well when the scalp is involved.

Nail fungal infections are resistant to any form of therapy. Many nonprescription remedies promise relief from this chronic problem. Here is a rule that you can take to the bank: no topical treatment currently on the market does anything to cure a fungal infection of the nail. If you are insistent on treating nail fungi, your only option is to use one of the systemic therapies for many months. Toenail infections take twelve to eighteen months of treatment; fingernail infections require about six months of therapy. Even if the infection clears, it may return shortly after treatment is discontinued. I spend a fair amount of time each week trying to dissuade patients from treating these types of infections.

Is treatment needed to prevent the infection from spreading to other family members? The organism can be spread from person to person, but the fungus is everywhere. If you eradicate it from your toes, there will be plenty of other places that can harbor the organism. There is no compelling rationale to treat fungal infections for public health reasons.

There are those who advocate prophylactic measures to prevent infections in those who are prone to them. These include loose-fitting footwear, absorbent socks, frequent changes of towels and clothing, and assiduous attention to drying the feet after showering. A moist environment plays some role in the promotion of fungal infections. If you assigned points for effectiveness, preventive measures would get one point and antifungal antibiotic therapy would get nine points. Others are more enthusiastic about these approaches to prevention. I have little enthusiasm for them after all the failures I have seen.

TINEA VERSICOLOR

As mentioned earlier, many fungal organisms live on the skin without symptoms. One of these is a fungus called *pityrosporum orbiculare*. When certain factors are present (warm, humid environment, pregnancy, and serious underlying diseases, are a few), the organism changes its structure and becomes a pathogen capable of causing a skin infection called tinea versicolor. Some people have a hereditary predisposition to this infection. Multiple family members may be affected. It gets its name because the lesions vary in color from white to brown to red. There is also a fine white scale that is loaded with organisms.

A typical appearance of tinea versicolor is a number of reticulated, round, flat, multicolored spots with a minimal overlying scale. The most common sites of involvement are the trunk and neck. The face and extremities may also be infected. The rash is usually asymptomatic. Summertime is the worst season for this kind of infection because the lesions look more obvious, this is true because as one tans, the lesions remain lighter and thus show up better.

The treatment of tinea versicolor is quite effective. You can treat yourself with an antidandruff shampoo used as a lotion over the affected area every other night for two weeks. This is messy and time consuming, but it can rid you of the infection, at least temporarily. Your doctor can prescribe a systemic antifungal agent that can clear the infection after only two doses. This is a cost- and time-effective means of treating this bothersome malady. The agent, ketoconazole, is used for serious systemic fungal diseases, and some are reluctant to risk the serious side effects to the liver for a trivial infection such as this. Two doses of anything can cause problems, but the chances are exceedingly small that you will have any adverse reactions with this tiny dose of ketoconazole.

Miscellaneous Lumps and Bumps

When you enter the world, your skin is usually perfect. It is soft, smooth, wrinkle free, and completely uniform. As you go through life, you acquire what one dermatologist I know calls "barnacles." These are harmless appendages that appear one day and never disappear. If you live long enough, I guarantee you that you will acquire one or more of these little nuisances. Try viewing them as counterparts to the wisdom you attain with years of experience. Unless you don't like the looks of these growths or they become irritated by your clothing or by your constant manipulation, there is no medical reason to have them removed.

SKIN TAGS

These fleshy papules often appear on the neck, in the underarm area, and in the groin. Anyone can develop them, but they are more common in overweight individuals. A few years ago, there was some concern that they occurred more often in people with polyps in the colon. This fear turned out to be unfounded. Skin tags and colonic polyps are both common, and it is not unusual for some people to have both conditions at the same time.

A skin tag is a brown, soft papule with a stalk that attaches it to the skin. Occasionally, the stalk can turn on itself and cut off the blood supply to the tag. This is an indication for removal of the affected lesion. If you wish to have these removed, they can be snipped flush with the skin, usually without local anesthesia.

SEBORRHEIC KERATOSIS

This benign growth appears as a flat, rough-surfaced pigmented papule. The edges are often lifted away from the skin surface, giving the lesion the appearance of being stuck on like a postage stamp. The color can vary from tan to dark blue-black, and there may be several different shades in the same lesion. They can appear anywhere but tend to concentrate on the trunk. African Americans have a variation of these keratoses on the face, which are tiny black papules with a rough surface.

Although seborrheic keratoses are completely harmless, they can sometimes mimic a melanoma, which, as you know, is a serious medical problem. There are times when the keratoses are so worrisome that diagnostic biopsies are performed to rule out skin cancer. This is a hard diagnosis for even experienced physicians. To be on the safe side, if there is even a remote concern on your part about one of your keratoses, allow your doctor to examine it. Patients will often apologize to me for "wasting my time" with unimportant skin growths like seborrheic keratoses. I love to tell them that the spot is benign and that if that relieves their concern, it was definitely worth the time and effort. If that doesn't persuade you to have a dermatologist look at your worrisome keratoses, perhaps this trade secret will do the trick: The most common skin problem that nondermatologist physicians send to me is a seborrheic keratosis that they think might be a melanoma. I am happy to give them a good report, and they are relieved that they do not have to make this kind of diagnosis without some help.

If you choose to have your seborrheic keratoses removed, there are several quick and effective ways to do it. My preference is to use an electric needle to gently burn them off. Others prefer to treat them by freezing them with liquid nitrogen. Either of these methods will remove the lesions. There is a 5% chance that the keratoses will recur. Some would advise you to have these lesions surgically excised with suture closure. This is far too involved and expensive for a simple therapeutic problem such as this. For those of you who are into self-treatment or cannot keep your hands off these crusty areas, there is no real harm in picking these growths off with your fingernails. They tend to recur more often this way, but there is no lasting harm done. However, if there is any doubt whatsoever that this could be something other than a seborrheic keratosis, don't manipulate it until your doctor has seen the lesion.

CHERRY ANGIOMA

These bright red spots appear in early adult life and increase in number with age. The name is quite apt since these look like minute cherries in the skin. They are bright red or slightly purple and are most common on the trunk but may appear on the face or extremities. It is common to have hundreds of these spots on the skin.

Cherry angiomas are composed of collections of small blood vessels in the upper part of the dermis. They may bleed if they are traumatized; otherwise, they are of little consequence. If you wish to have some of these removed, a quick and simple method is to anesthetize them and to cauterize the vessels with an electric needle. Expect a scar after such a procedure.

LENTIGO

A lentigo is a brown spot that occurs on chronically sun-exposed parts of the skin, particularly on the backs of the hands, the upper back, and the face. It is also known as an age spot, although it can appear relatively early in life. Another moniker is liver spot, presumably because it sometimes has the brown-red hue of liver. It has no relationship with any liver disorder. Lentigos are uniformly tan-brown. They have a star-shaped appearance with jagged edges, and they are always perfectly flat.

Since sun exposure is an important etiologic factor, you can minimize further lentigos by protecting your skin from the sun. It is more difficult to remove these lesions than to prevent them. If you choose to have them treated, there are bleaching creams on the market that claim to lighten these spots. At best, these do a mediocre job of fading lentigos. It takes many months of continuous therapy. The result is usually only a slight change in the lesion but a considerable lightening of your pocketbook. Other methods of treating these spots are described in chapter 8.

CYST

A cyst arising in the skin is a closed sac containing keratin protein. When the protein drains, it is cheesy and foul smelling. It may arise as an outpouching from a hair follicle, known as a follicular cyst or epidermoid cyst. It may also occur just below the epidermis as a small kernel called a milium.

Epidermoid cysts appear as deep-seated, flesh-colored nodules. They sometimes have a prominent pore coming through to the surface. They may appear anywhere that there are hair follicles and are common on the scalp and back. Milia are often on the face and may be multiple. They occur as asymptomatic tiny white papules.

Most epidermoid cysts sit silently under the skin and are barely visible. These should be left alone. You may wish to have an epidermoid cyst removed if it drains its contents frequently or becomes inflamed or infected. Surgical excision is the most effective way to remove the cyst permanently. If it is drained of its contents without removing the cyst wall, it usually recurs. Milia are purely a cosmetic problem. They rarely become infected or inflamed. Incising and draining them will often cure them.

Hives

There are few skin diseases more frustrating for both the patient and the physician than hives (urticaria). We all want to be able to pinpoint the source of a problem and set about to eliminate that cause. Unfortunately, this is difficult or impossible in most cases of hives. In the quest for the answer, many will disrupt their lives to the point where it would have been easier to live with the skin problem. It reminds me of the Gene Hackman movie in which the character destroys his house looking for an eavesdropping device that is supposedly monitoring his activities. Not only does he not detect the bugging apparatus, but he is left with no floors or walls. This cautionary tale is appropriate when discussing hives. Sometimes the cause is too obscure to spend the time and effort that can scramble one's life.

Hives are distinctive and should not be too difficult for you to diagnose when you see them. They are raised, red, swollen plaques (wheals) with sharply defined margins surrounded by a red or white halo. They may cover most of the body, or there may be only a few small wheals. The lesions can come up within minutes and always disappear within twenty-four hours. If a given lesion remains unchanged for more than one day, you probably do not have hives. Urticaria is often described as "traveling around." What is happening is th old wheals quickly disappear and new ones in different locations take their place.

The classification of urticaria has been arbitrarily divided into an acute and chronic phase. If the episode is less than six weeks old, it is considered acute. If the hives keep appearing beyond six weeks, it is classified as chronic. This is an important distinction since once someone has gone longer than 6 weeks without a cause being determined, the odds of uncovering the source of the problem are less than one in five. The underlying problems that lead to hives are divided into six categories:

- Medication reactions*

- Infections*

- Rheumatic diseases

- Neoplastic diseases (cancer)

- Foods, food dyes, and food preservatives

- Psychogenic urticaria

The top two on the list have been starred because they are the most common causes of acute urticaria, and they are the easiest to pin down. If you develop hives for the first time, try to reconstruct the previous fourteen days of your life. Have you started taking any new medications? Have you had an illness that caused you to run a fever? Has there been any illness that has affected several members of your household? If you have answered yes to any of these questions, you may have figured out for yourself the reason you developed hives.

The other possibilities on the list must be investigated by your physician. There is no urgency in doing this; most cases of hives regress by themselves within a few days without therapy. If this happens with you, you do not need to go through the exercise of ruling out unusual causes of your problem. If the rash is symptomatic, you can use an over-the-counter antihistamine such as diphenhydramine or chlorpheniramine. Both of these drugs work by blocking the action of histamine in the skin. They are only effective if they are in your system when the histamine arrives in the skin. If you take one of these pills after each episode of hives begins, you will always be too late; the medicine must be taken before the wheals evolve. These drugs are effective antihistamines but they are also sedating. Many are caught with a dilemma of needing to take the medicine throughout the day but not being able to function at work because of the drowsiness that antihistamines cause.

If your hives continue for more than a week in spite of full-dose antihistamines or if you cannot tolerate the side effects of these medications, consult with your doctor. She will take a detailed history and do a limited physical examination to try to detect the cause of your hives. This work-up may include some blood tests. She may then prescribe one of the newer nonsedating, prescription antihistamines—be prepared to pay up to two dollars per pill for these drugs. She may also give you additional medications to slow down the process.

Some drugs can cause hives to worsen, even if they are not the direct reason they broke out initially. These include aspirin, other nonsteroidal anti-inflammatory medications such as ibuprofen, and codeine. If you are taking one of these medications, your hives might improve if you switch to something else.

If six weeks pass and you are still getting new outbreaks, your doctor may perform a wide-ranging evaluation to find the cause of your problem. As I mentioned above, don't count on a definitive answer unless there is some clue that she uncovers in taking your medical history or performing a physical examination. If you feel completely well and have chronic urticaria, it is unusual to come to the right answer even with many laboratory tests. Here is another trade secret: If your doctor orders more than ten different tests, she is going on a fishing expedition. Not very many fish are caught that way.

If a complete analysis of your case has been concluded and the source of your rash has not been determined, your doctor may suggest that you consult an allergist. Many of these physicians are exceptional detectives; they can uncover occult allergens that others may have missed. You may be subjected to very demanding diet modifications and other changes in your environment as a part of the program. Remember the parable about the movie character who knocked down his house. Try to avoid the same sort of thing happening to you as your allergist seeks to sort out the mystery. I would rather have hives and be able to eat what I like rather than live on a diet of boiled chicken and rice for a few months. You may have to make a similar value judgment. Foods and food additives are an uncommon cause of chronic urticaria.

In many people, urticaria is a psychosomatic disorder, listed above as "psychogenic." This is a diagnosis that one falls to after other possibilities have been dismissed. If your hives occur during stressful times in your life, you may be able to cure yourself by many of the same relaxation strategies discussed in the section on atopic dermatitis.

Itch

A most distressing symptom that plagues everyone at some time is itch, or pruritus. I knew a highly successful businessman with everything in the world to live for who committed suicide because he could no longer stand the persistent itch that troubled him for years. Itchiness can ruin your life just as harshly as cancer, drug addiction, or mental illness. In most instances, pruritus is associated with an identifiable skin disorder such as atopic dermatitis or hives. In many situations, however, there is no obvious reason why the skin is itchy. It is this circumstance that is addressed in the following section. I also discuss a type of localized itch without an obvious etiology, pruritus ani (anal itching).

There are three categories of conditions that cause an itch without an obvious rash: occult skin disease, manifested only by itching; internal disease, with pruritus as one manifestation; and psychogenic pruritus.

OCCULT SKIN DISORDER

Many skin conditions have subtle clinical findings. If you examine a sample of the skin under a microscope, there might be some clue to the diagnosis. The most common cause of pruritus without an obvious eruption is dry skin (xerosis). (For a complete discussion of xerosis and what to do about it, see chapter 3.) This is really a functional disorder rather than an anatomic abnormality. The skin does not hold water well but it often looks entirely normal. If you itch mostly in the winter, start lubricating your skin twice daily and cut back on bathing. Your pruritus may disappear within a week. A special name has been given to this condition, "winter itch." If you itch and it is wintertime, you have it until proven otherwise.

INTERNAL DISEASE

Several serious systemic illnesses may affect the skin. Generalized itching is often the cutaneous manifestation. These include end-stage kidney disease, obstructive liver disease, AIDS, certain cancers, several endocrine abnormalities, and blood disorders including iron deficiency anemia. With few exceptions, the itch is preceded by the illness that causes it. In almost all of these situations, the underlying diagnosis has long since been established before the onset of pruritus. I am emphasizing this so that you will not rush to your doctor for an evaluation at the first inkling that you might be itchy. If you feel well other than your itch, try a little skin lubrication first.

PSYCHOGENIC PRURITUS

A recurrent theme throughout this book has been the role your emotional state plays in the determination of your skin's health. Generalized itching occurs regularly in people who are in the throes of an emotional upheaval. As I noted in the section on atopic dermatitis, those who have a genetic predisposition for atopy will flare more when stressed. They do so because the skin is itchy and they scratch. The scratching leads to the eruption. In many cases of psychogenic pruritus, this atopic predisposition is present. The affected individuals have not scratched vigorously enough to produce a rash.

The management of generalized pruritus is similar to that for atopic dermatitis, with a few exceptions. Topical corticosteroids are not very effective in the absence of an obvious dermatitis. Hydrocortisone 1% cream is harmless, but its effects are minimal in this situation. If an internal cause of the pruritus can be determined, successful treatment of that problem usually clears the itch as well. One exception to that rule is in the case of the person who must be dialyzed because his kidneys have failed. In some of these unfortunate people, dialysis will improve their physical health but will greatly exacerbate the itch.

ANAL ITCH

One of the most exasperating and embarrassing symptoms is an itchy anus, or pruritus ani. If your neck itches, you don't hesitate to scratch it, even in the middle of crowd of strangers. Very few people would dare scratch their rectums in public, however. Only the most understanding spouse would condone an episode of wild scratching of the rectum, punctuating an otherwise uneventful dinner with the family.

This symptom is very common. The absence of scratching attests to the extraordinary will power and social grace of millions of people who are afflicted with this condition.

There are numerous identifiable causes of pruritus ani. These include pinworm infestations, yeast infections of the large bowel, hemorrhoids, and skin diseases such as psoriasis and seborrheic dermatitis. Unfortunately, these account for only a minority of cases. In most people, the itch is the final common symptom caused by many mild irritants, including feces, toilet tissue, clothing, and sweat. Since there are so many possible contributing factors, a shotgun approach to management is often used:

- Optimize anal hygiene. After each bowel movement, wash the area around the anus with a water-soluble cleanser. Avoid harsh soaps. Another option is to use premoistened pads. Apply a drying powder at least once a day; a good time to do this is after showering.

- At the first hint of itching, apply hydrocortisone 1% cream. This can be used two or three times a day if necessary. Do not use stronger corticosteroid preparations in the perianal area. They can cause skin thinning, which will add to your problems.

- If you notice that there is fecal leakage onto the skin between bowel movements, place a wisp of cotton over the anal opening to catch this material.

- Hard stool can irritate the anal skin. Try drinking a tablespoon of a stool softener such as Metamucil in juice twice daily. If this gives you excess gas, cut the dose in half.

- Try sitz baths in tepid water, which can be soothing and can gently cleanse the skin.

If these techniques do not improve the itch substantially in one month, you should consult your doctor. A simple test such as anoscopy will uncover whether hemorrhoids are the root of your trouble. Hemorrhoids secrete an irritating mucous that worsens anal itch. If you note bright red blood on the toilet tissue after wiping and if there is a moist feel to the perianal area all the time, hemorrhoids may be responsible.

Psoriasis

Psoriasis is a chronic skin disease that affects 1% to 3% of the world's population. Many are not even aware that they have a skin disorder.

They think the scaly spots are dry skin, an irritation from clothing, or a reaction to friction. For these people, psoriasis is far from a "heart-breaking" disease. Many others are troubled by persistent, unsightly scaly patches. They can be a cosmetic embarrassment, can be itchy, and can be associated with a disabling form of arthritis.

The pathogenesis of psoriasis is complicated and not completely clear. There is definitely a genetic component in many cases. About 30% of affected individuals report a family member with psoriasis. There also seems to be immune dysregulation that leads to skin inflammation and increased cellular growth of the epidermis. As with many of the other conditions that affect the skin, there is a psychosomatic component to psoriasis. Stress can cause extreme flares of an otherwise inactive condition. The net result is that the skin becomes thicker and scalier.

Any skin site can be affected. The most common areas of involvement are those that are exposed to mild trauma, such as the elbows and knees. Many psoriatics develop patches after skin injuries; for example, a person may undergo an operation and get psoriasis in the wound scar. The scalp is another target area of thick, scaly plaques. Perhaps the minimal trauma associated with combing the hair is enough to set off the pathologic process. The nails are frequently involved as well.

A typical lesion of psoriasis is a well-defined red, scaly plaque, or papule. If the scale is removed, a small bleeding point is noted. The nails can be grossly distorted. There is scale under the nail plate, and the plate itself may also be disfigured. Careful inspection of the plate may reveal tiny pits. This is one of the diagnostic hallmarks of psoriasis and is an important clue in people with only a few scaly skin lesions.

Once you develop psoriasis, you are seldom completely cured of it. However, there may be long periods when little or no activity will be evident. I have cared for patients who had twenty-year breaks between attacks. If your doctor makes this diagnosis, it is not a reason for despair. There are many effective remedies; even without aggressive treatment, it is quite likely that you will be like millions of others and have only minimal disease.

If you decide to treat your psoriasis, your state of mind and degree of motivation will be extremely important. Those who do best with treatment look at the disease as the enemy in a long guerrilla war where many small skirmishes will be fought. If you let up, the guerrillas will come down from the hills and take over the major cities (your skin). You will need to continue the treatment month after month to keep your skin looking as good as possible. If you let up, the disease might flare in just a few days. If you can adopt the attitude that your psoriasis treatment is a normal part of your daily routine, like showering and using cosmetics, you will have a good chance at keeping even serious cases at bay. Don't go into this war looking for a quick victory; it does not happen with psoriasis. With that pep talk in mind, here are some of the steps you can take, even before consulting with a dermatologist.

For very mild cases of psoriasis, hydrocortisone 1% ointment applied twice daily may decrease the severity of individual lesions. Psoriasis is not a particularly steroid-responsive condition, so don't expect too much from this approach. One way to increase the efficacy of hydrocortisone in the therapy for localized plaques is to apply a piece of polyethylene wrap (like Saran Wrap) over the cream at bedtime. Remove the wrap in the morning.

Psoriasis often responds to coal tar preparations. I am sure that the thought of applying thick black ointment to your skin does not sound particularly enticing. Newer, cosmetically acceptable products such as Estar or Psorigel are available, making this therapeutic alternative acceptable. The medications are applied at night and washed off in the morning. Another way to apply tar is in the form of a tar-based bath oil. This is added to running bath water as the tub is filled. You bathe in this emulsion for fifteen to thirty minutes. The only problem with this approach is that the tub can acquire an impressive black ring. If you use tar, be careful when you go out in the sun. Tar will make your skin more sensitive to even small amounts of ultraviolet light.

There are a few problems that you may encounter when using tars. They can stain your skin and clothing, so it is important that they be applied sparingly at night and removed completely when you shower in the morning. Tars can also plug the pores and produce inflammation of the hair follicles (folliculitis). If this happens, stop using the tar for a few days. Treat the folliculitis by scrubbing with antibacterial soaps twice daily. Try the tars again after the lesions are improved. If the folliculitis recurs, you may have to abandon this form of treatment.

Psoriasis is one of the few skin conditions that improves with sunlight exposure. This is the only time anybody ever hears a dermatologist recommend that a patient intentionally sunbathe. Ultraviolet light therapy alone may completely clear your psoriasis, and your skin may stay clear for months afterward in many instances. This type of treatment must be approached as a carefully planned regimen, not as an excuse to sit outdoors every so often. In order for ultraviolet therapy to work, you must perform the treatment at least three times a week until it clears up. Only those skin sites that are directly exposed to the light will have a chance to improve. Sitting out on the lawn, fully clothed, during your lunch hour will not get the job done. In most parts of the country, summertime is the only practical time of the year to do this type of treatment. However, if you push this in the summer, you may stay clear through the winter months.

If you can arrange the time and place for sunlight exposure, start slowly at ten to fifteen minutes per side. This should be done between 11:00 A.M. and 2:00 P.M. to take advantage of the peak time for ultraviolet rays. Increase the dose of light by five minutes every two treatments until a given exposure causes you to barely turn pink. That is your dose (amount of time in the sun) from that point forward. If your face does not have psoriatic lesions, which is the usual case, wear strong sunscreens there to prevent unnecessary sun damage. Do not put sunscreens on your psoriatic plaques. They will block out the light that your skin needs to help your psoriasis.

In the winter, you may be tempted to use your handy neighborhood tanning salon to keep the treatment going. This will not help you since the wavelength of light emitted from these bulbs is not what you need. (See chapter 4 for a complete discussion of tanning salons.)

There are shampoos specially formulated to remove the scale and calm the redness of psoriatic plaques on the scalp. These are extremely helpful and should be used daily if necessary. They are discussed in detail in the section on seborrheic dermatitis.

Psoriatic nails can be greatly disfigured. Topical treatments, including ultraviolet light, do not work in improving this situation. Cosmetic cover-ups are the best way to handle this difficult problem. Several effective strategies are discussed in chapter 8.

Again, I return to the area of stress management and psoriasis control. There is a popular psoriasis treatment facility at the Dead Sea in Israel. People from throughout the world come to this place for four to six weeks to "take the cure." The proponents claim that the salt water and the strong ultraviolet light make this program successful. Perhaps that is true. I suspect that even more important is that the person is removed from a tension-filled environment and transported to an idyllic setting, where he can lounge on the beach for days at a time, without a care in the world. You don't need a trip to the Dead Sea to get the same benefit. Find the spot that is right for you and drop down there for a couple of weeks. Your psoriasis may improve dramatically.

If these techniques do not improve your psoriasis sufficiently, a consultation with a dermatologist is the next step. There are many treatment options that she has that can substantially improve or even clear your skin. Note that as the aggressiveness of the treatment increases, so do the potential side effects of the therapy. You need to decide in advance what risks you are willing to take to achieve success. If you are concerned about medication toxicity to the point where you are not willing to take substantial risks, you need to inform your doctor so that an appropriate program can be designed. Lifestyle issues must be addressed as well. If you work all day and cannot spare the time to come to the doctor's office for treatments on a regular basis, home-based therapies are probably more appropriate for you. As I stated in chapter 1, your doctor is there to serve you; what she thinks is best might not suit your needs. She needs to know exactly what you think. What is mild to her may be devastating to you. You may feel that even a small amount of skin involvement warrants aggressive treatment. For you, this is the right choice. Let your feelings be known. Here are some alternatives that your dermatologist may discuss with you.

POTENT TOPICAL CORTICOSTEROIDS

As mentioned in the section on atopic dermatitis, there are several grades of topical corticosteroids. Since psoriasis is not sensitive to these agents, often only the strongest of these preparations will work. For localized disease, these medications can substantially improve the appearance of the skin, but they seldom completely clear the lesions. For generalized psoriasis, it becomes impractical and expensive to smear these creams over such a large area twice daily. A tube of one of these products may cost fifty dollars and may last less than a week if used over much of the body.

ANTHRALIN

This chemical is related to coal tar and is used extensively in hospitals in Europe for thick plaques of psoriasis. It is not as popular in the United States because it is incredibly messy. Since very few patients with psoriasis in the United States are hospitalized for psoriasis treatment and since few people are happy about messing up their homes with this product, it is seldom used.

Anthralin does improve psoriasis if you can stick with the treatment for several weeks at a time. It is particularly useful in localized thick plaques on the elbows and knees. The medication is applied as an ointment or paste and left in place for ten to thirty minutes. It is then washed off with liquid soap. This sounds simple, but the agent does not always come off the skin completely. It also temporarily stains the skin a red-brown color and may irritate the skin surrounding the psoriatic plaques that are treated. If you get it on your clothing, it is impossible to remove.

UVB PHOTOTHERAPY

If sunlight works for you in the summer, your doctor may suggest that he administer ultraviolet light to you during the winter months. This will involve going into a light box for a few minutes three to five times per week. Many people get substantial improvement after twenty to thirty treatments. This treatment makes you a slave to the light box. If you go away on a winter vacation, the missed treatment sessions may set you back substantially. Although each treatment is short, busy dermatologists may have many people using the box. So even though you do not need to see the doctor each time you get a treatment, you may have to wait in line to use the facility. If you have a tight schedule, this could be a pitfall.

PHOTOCHEMOTHERAPY

An effective way to use ultraviolet light in psoriasis is to combine it with a medication that is activated by the light to work against the psoriatic plaques. This is the principle behind photochemotherapy, or PUVA, an acronym that stands for psoralen, the drug which is taken internally, and uva, the type of ultraviolet light that activates the psoralen. The drug is taken two hours before exposure to the light. Treatments are given two or three times a week until a remission is achieved. At that point a maintenance program is instituted to keep the skin clear. This may be as infrequently as once or twice a month.

The main advantages of PUVA are that it works even in severe forms of psoriasis and you do not have to apply ointments day after day to keep the skin looking near normal. The big disadvantage of this form of therapy is that chronic PUVA therapy will make you prone to skin cancer and premature aging of the skin. If you have bad psoriasis now, what your skin may look like ten years in the future may not seem important. It is something to consider, however, before you agree to this treatment program. Photochemotherapy is an expensive way to treat psoriasis, although many insurance plans cover much of the cost. The psoralen pills may cost you up to fifteen dollars a week; the light treatments are thirty to forty dollars per session.

METHOTREXATE

The gold standard against which all treatments for psoriasis are measured is methotrexate. This is the most effective therapy that is available. It can clear your psoriasis and keep it clear for as long as you continue to take the medication. If this is so great, why doesn't everyone with psoriasis skip the lesser treatments and go right to this drug? There is a one-word answer to this question: toxicity. This drug can affect the liver, particularly in those who have some liver damage already. If you enjoy your beer or liquor or you have had hepatitis, methotrexate is a bad choice for you.

If you and your doctor determine that you are a good candidate for this medication, a battery of laboratory tests will be run as a baseline to compare against in the future. If any abnormalities do surface, these usually revert to normal when the drug is stopped. Unfortunately, blood tests are not always an accurate mirror of liver damage; therefore, liver biopsies will be required every one to three years to better assess the status of your liver.

Methotrexate is an easy drug to take. You take the medication only one day a week. On that day, you may be nauseated or feel fatigued. This can be minimized by ingesting the medication at bedtime. Many people need a high dose at the start of treatment but require only small maintenance doses once they have improved. If you stop the treatment altogether, expect to see your psoriasis return within a few weeks.

ETRETINATE

If you have severe psoriasis and cannot take methotrexate, etretinate is another effective systemic therapy to consider. It is most beneficial in two unusual psoriasis variants: pustular psoriasis and psoriasis that makes you red and scaly all over (erythrodermic psoriasis). It also works in the relief of the common type of disease, but the response is slow and often incomplete. This is another synthetic derivative of vitamin A. It is similar to isotretinoin, which is discussed in the section on acne. This expensive drug must be taken daily and may add up to a cost of over two hundred dollars a month. As with all the other remedies, the drug's effects do not carry over when it is discontinued.

The side effects of etretinate are more bothersome than dangerous. Dry skin and lips occur to some extent in everyone on this medication. Headaches, hair loss, muscle aches and peeling of the palms and soles are also fairly common. Some develop fragile skin, and even a small bump will cause it to shear and it will heal slowly. Some people complain of a sticky feeling on the skin. One disastrous adverse effect associated with etretinate use is significant malformations in children born to women who become pregnant while on this drug. Since it stays in the body indefinitely, women who have any intention of ever having children cannot take this drug until their childbearing years are behind them.

CYCLOSPORINE

The newest addition to the arsenal against psoriasis is the drug used to prevent organ transplant rejection. This medication works extremely well, even in the worst cases of psoriasis. However, it is also the most toxic of all the possible treatments. For this reason, only those with life-ruining disease for whom all other options have failed are candidates for this treatment. Many dermatologists would prefer to have a consultant at a medical center administer this drug. So you may have to travel some distance to have access to this form of therapy.

Seborrheic Dermatitis

An itchy scalp is never going to kill you, but it certainly can make life unpleasant. The most common cause of scalp pruritus is seborrhea. If there is scale without redness, it is called dandruff. If redness of the scalp coexists with the excess scale, it bears the name seborrheic dermatitis. Either variant can produce symptoms. There is much controversy about the cause of this problem. Some believe that a yeast organism that lives on the scalp is the main culprit. Others contend that the yeast is along for the ride but is not the immediate cause of the condition. Seborrhea occurs in areas that have many sebaceous glands; these include the scalp, the central part of the face, and the chest. Seborrhea is rarely a problem before puberty, the time when oil glands become active. Some have concluded that sebum secreted from these glands is playing a role in the development of the disease. One other peculiar finding adds to the mystery of this disease; people with the neurologic disease Parkinson's syndrome have severe and recalcitrant seborrheic dermatitis. Could there be a connection between the defect in the brain and the skin condition? No one knows for sure.

The typical case of dandruff features intermittent scalp itching and increased scaling. When there is inflammation as well, the scalp is red and may be crusty. A similar process may occur on the face. People mistake the redness and scale of this disease for dryness or allergy to cosmetics. There are several clues to direct you toward the diagnosis of seborrheic dermatitis. These include scaling and redness in the central part of the eyebrows, redness and itching at the corner of the wing of the nose, where it meets the upper lip, and scaling of the upper eyelids. Occasionally there is also redness and scaling of the chin and chest; this occurs between the nipples in men and under the breasts in women.

In most instances, you can successfully care for your seborrhea problem without the assistance of a physician. You need to regard this as something that will not be cured but that can be well controlled by routine measures. Don't get frustrated if the condition returns repeatedly. View it as a challenge to suppress it as quickly as possible.

Anti-seborrheic shampoos contain ingredients that remove scale, reduce inflammation, and decrease epidermal proliferation that leads to excess scale initially. They also contain strong detergents to remove sebum from the scalp and hair. There is no clearly superior ingredient that is best for everyone. Try different types to see which one you like best. Here are some of your choices:

- Selenium sulfide (Selsun, Exsel). This works well but has a distinctive smell that may be objectionable if you are sensitive to such things.

- Zinc pyrithione (Head and Shoulders, Zincon, ZNP). Products with this ingredient are widely used because they are effective and because of extensive advertising. If you have facial seborrhea, consider ZNP. It is in bar form and can be used as a shampoo on the scalp and as a scrub on the face.

- Tar (T/Gel, Ionil-T, Denorex). Old-fashioned heavy, foul-smelling tar shampoos have given way to fairly acceptable products. If you have white or light blond hair, consider another alternative; tar shampoos may stain these hair colors a muddy yellow-brown. One tar-based shampoo claims that it is superior because it tingles when applied to the scalp. The agent that produces the tingling is an inactive ingredient. Don't buy a shampoo simply because it tingles.

- Salicylic acid-sulfur (Sebulex, Ionil Plus, VanSeb). Many people prefer this type of shampoo because the active ingredients break the bonds that hold scale on the scalp. These shampoos are fine but they are not any more effective than the other types at decreasing scaliness.

For most people, daily shampooing with one of the medicated shampoos is sufficient to control the problem. For some reason, the dermatitis on the face and trunk may also improve by regular shampooing. The more frequently you cleanse your scalp, the better your results. Some people shampoo infrequently because of a concern for excess dryness. If your hair feels dry, use a conditioner. What you regard as a dry scalp may be inadequately treated seborrhea itself.

Take your time when you shampoo. A quick wash and rinse does not allow enough time for the agents to work on the scalp. For best results, shampoo and rinse once, then shampoo and relax for three or four minutes while the shampoo does its job. To remove all remaining dirt and oil, the final rinse should be vigorous.

If shampooing alone doesn't control your problem, try hydrocortisone 1% lotion. Apply it after each shampoo and, if needed, again at bedtime. This will reduce the scalp inflammation and flaking. Although lotions are watery, your hair may feel a little greasy after applying these preparations.

If, after trying all of these methods, your seborrheic dermatitis is still active, it is time to consult your dermatologist. Perhaps your scalp condition is caused by something else. Stronger medicine may be needed to control the problem. She may use more potent cortisone preparations to bring the condition under control. If she gives you one of these agents, do not use it on your face for more than two weeks without a one-week break. Some people do well with a topical antifungal cream. This presumably controls the yeasts that may be one of the causes of seborrhea. This is very safe medicine; however, do not expect it to work much better than a topical corticosteroid like hydrocortisone.

Warts

Warts are benign tumors caused by a family of viruses that infect the skin. Even after the virus is gone, the tumor may remain. Conversely, the virus may lay dormant for years without ever producing a tumor (wart). Warts may occur at any age but are most common between ages twelve and sixteen. They spread from person to person and by auto-inoculation (spread from one site on your skin to another site by scratching, and so forth).

In part due to different virus subtypes and in part due to the location of the virus inoculation, there are several different ways that a wart can appear:

- Common warts. These start as small, flesh-colored papules that over several months become larger raised, rough-surfaced lesions. Occasionally there are tiny black dots in the papules, which are the capillaries supplying the blood to the warts. Common warts are most frequently found on the hands but may occur elsewhere.

- Flat warts. These lesions often appear in clusters on the face, neck, and hands. They are minute, flesh-colored, flat-topped bumps that look identical to one another.

- Filiform warts. These usually appear as solitary, soft, thin, finger-like growths on the face and neck. Adults get these more often than children.

- Plantar warts. These are the warts that occur on the bottoms of the feet (the plantar surface). This is often misconstrued as *planter's* warts, a disease mistakenly thought to be endemic in farmers. Plantar warts are sometimes painful because of the trauma of walking on them. They appear as firm papules with a rough surface, often in pressure points directly under the bones of the foot.

- Genital warts (condyloma accuminata). Warts that grow in warm, moist places such as under the foreskin on the penis, in the vagina, or around the rectum develop into soft vegetating, grapelike clusters. Small, solitary lesions may also appear as white papules.

Wart treatment is a real adventure. When you start out, you never know what the outcome will be. In one person, a placebo therapy may eliminate the warts in days. In another person with the same type of lesions, years of effort may be expended as the lesions proliferate like mushrooms. Literally scores of treatment methods have been touted as effective in eradicating warts. A good rule to remember is that if there are more than five different treatments for a problem, none of them is likely to be a cure-all. Warts are unique in that more aggressive therapy is not necessarily more successful. Whatever treatment you pick has about a 70% chance of causing a remission. This includes watchful waiting without any treatment whatsoever.

The therapeutic options listed below are the ones most commonly used. If a strange-sounding alternative to these approaches works for you, go for it. None of these treatments kills the virus that causes the wart to grow. They eradicate the tumor itself. If the virus remains in the skin, it is possible that your wart will return. None of these methods goes deep into the skin; this is not necessary since warts do not have deep roots to provide them nourishment. They reside in the epidermis only. Many of these techniques physically remove the epidermal layer, and the wart comes off with it.

One word of caution is in order before you set out to treat your own warts. If you are not absolutely certain that a given skin lesion is a wart, defer therapy until your physician confirms the diagnosis. I have seen several melanomas treated as warts for months before the correct diagnosis was finally made. This major disaster can be avoided by getting a professional opinion.

CRYOTHERAPY

This method is usually done with liquid nitrogen, an extremely cold substance. It causes a localized frostbite that produces a blister. The roof of the blister contains the whole epidermis, including the wart. When it sloughs, the wart falls off with it. This treatment is uncomfortable, and the ensuing blisters can remain sore for several days. The skin site may turn white after healing, because the freezing can damage melanocytes that make skin pigment. Several treatments are often necessary, and your doctor will probably schedule them one to three weeks apart to allow one treatment to work before the next is undertaken.

The liquid nitrogen is applied in one of two ways: a cotton-tipped swab is dipped in a canister and then applied to the wart or a spray apparatus attached to an insulated bottle filled with liquid nitrogen is used to spray the substance on the wart. The second approach is faster and gets the wart to a colder temperature, but it hurts a little more than the cotton-tipped swap method. It takes only a few seconds to treat the average wart, whichever technique is utilized.

CANTHARIDIN

Medicine meets entomology when physicians use cantharidin for warts. This is an extract from a blister beetle. The medicine is a sticky liquid that is painted directly onto the wart. When applied it produces a blister much like liquid nitrogen does. A piece of tape is placed over the site and is left untouched for twenty-four hours. This is a good treatment for children because there is no discomfort at the time of application. The area does get sore later in the day, however. One technical problem with cantharidin is that there is no way to predict whether a blister will actually form. With cryotherapy, if you freeze hard enough, there will be a reaction; this is not the case with cantharidin. Your doctor will probably ask you to return for additional treatment if a blister is not forthcoming within two or three days.

ELECTROSURGERY

This technique involves an electric needle that chars the wart and produces a split between the epidermis and the underlying skin. Like cryotherapy, when the epidermis is removed, the wart comes off with it. This method is somewhat more involved because local anesthesia is needed. After the site has been numbed, the electric needle is applied to the wart. As the treatment progresses, you may smell something burning; it's your wart being burnt. When the lesion is suitably desiccated, a sharp instrument called a curette is used to scrape off the dead tissue, including the wart.

This method has the advantage of being a one-treatment approach; you walk out the door without your wart. There is, however, no guarantee that the virus is eliminated from your skin. You may get the wart back within weeks. The main problem with this method is it leaves a scar. If it is on your hand, you may not mind, but if the wart is on your face you may want to consider methods that don't leave a mark.

KERATOLYTIC THERAPY

The best choice for home therapy is one of the agents that peels the wart away. Many of these strong keratolytic preparations used to be available by prescription only. Now, most can be purchased over the counter. Look for a product containing at least 15% salicylic acid and 15% lactic acid in a liquid base. These agents are particularly useful in children because they are painless to apply. They work slowly but there is no great rush to remove most warts. This method is valuable for plantar warts, particularly in active people. If your plantar wart is treated with cryotherapy or electrosurgery, you may be hobbled for a week or more. Keratolytic agents should not slow you down at all. On the other hand, if your plantar warts are painful and it is difficult for you to remain active because of this, this slow method may not be aggressive enough for your needs.

If you choose to use keratolytics, reserve some time every night to perform the treatment. Soak the wart in water for a few minutes to soften up the tissue. Then paint the medication on with the applicator that comes with the bottle. The material dries shortly after application. Every few days, pare off the old wart with an emery board or with a pumice stone. If irritation develops, stop therapy for a few days. This treatment may take a few months, depending on the thickness of the wart.

If all of this rigmarole is not what you have in mind for a little wart on your foot, try a salicylic acid plaster, which can be purchased at the foot-care counter in the supermarket. Apply the pad containing the acid to the wart and leave it in place for three to five days. After removing the pad, pare the white, softened top of the wart and apply another pad. This method has two advantages. There is minimal time spent on treatment, and there is a protective pad on the wart that might otherwise be painful to walk on. The disadvantage is that it is a slow method. If you are not in a rush, it is an excellent and inexpensive alternative.

IRRITANTS

There are times when there are so many warts that it becomes almost impossible to treat the lesions one at a time. This is particularly true of flat warts, where there may be hundreds of tiny lesions. Your body's immune system can rid itself of warts if it can be stimulated. In some instances, when a wart becomes inflamed the body turns on its immune mechanisms and eradicates not only the inflamed lesions but all the other warts as well. This is the rationale behind applying substances to irritate the warts. You might try the acne medicine benzoyl peroxide 10% gel, for this purpose. Apply it at least twice daily until redness and scaling develop. At this point, cut back treatment frequency to once daily. Give this method at least six weeks to succeed. If the warts are not disappearing after eight to ten weeks, you may need to progress to another approach.

PODOPHYLLIN

The most widely used medication for genital warts is podophyllin. It will only work in lesions on mucous membranes like the vagina and anus. It is not effective in genital warts on the shaft of the penis or the skin outside of the vagina. Your doctor will apply the dark brown liquid to the warts every one to two weeks until the lesions regress. A few hours later, you must bath or shower to remove the chemical. It often takes months of therapy to cure the warts in these locations. There is no discomfort when the medicine is applied, but the treated sites can be sore for days after each application. This drug should not be used on a pregnant woman because it may harm the developing fetus.

LASER SURGERY

An example of technology searching for diseases is laser therapy for recalcitrant warts. You should look at the laser as a very expensive electric needle. It does nothing qualitatively different from what electrosurgery does, which is burn the wart. The advantage of the laser is that the depth of penetration can be more closely monitored. Another technical advantage in treating warts around the fingernail is that the nail plate can be removed easily with the laser. In this way, any wart under the plate can be removed. The major disadvantage of laser therapy is that the cost is way out of proportion to the severity of the lesion treated. Even wealthy people with good health insurance might be taken aback by a $750 charge for removal of a single plantar wart.

The method is similar to that used in electrosurgery. The site is anesthetized locally. The laser burns the surface of the wart, then it is scraped off with a curette. Postoperative pain is somewhat less with a laser because the small nerve endings are sealed by the laser beam. You are likely to have a scar after this procedure.

INTERFERON

The use of interferon is another example of high technology treating low-tech diseases. Interferon is a naturally occurring protein that has been reproduced in the laboratory. It keeps certain cancers from multiplying and may have similar effects in virally-induced tumors. The medication is mostly used in extensive genital warts. It is injected three times weekly for three weeks. The discomfort of the injections is minimal, but most people get flulike symptoms later during the day of treatment.

The advantage of this technique is that there is no cutting or other surgical manipulation of the lesions. The main disadvantages are that you must return for nine treatments without a guarantee that it will cure your warts, and a therapeutic course costs hundreds of dollars.

BLEOMYCIN

Another injectable form of therapy that will cost less and may work as well is bleomycin. This is a drug used to treat cancer in doses substantially higher than those used to treat warts. The medicine is injected directly into the wart. The only major pitfall of using bleomycin is that it is incredibly painful to undergo this injection. I have made grown men cry with this therapy. After the treatment, the wart may remain painful for several days. Small warts may require only one treatment. Larger lesions or those in difficult-to-treat locations usually need several injections.

Herpes Infections

Over the past two decades, herpes infections have become synonymous with the sexual revolution, promiscuity, and a rise in the incidence of sexually transmitted diseases. In fact, long before there was a sexual revolution, virtually everyone was exposed to herpes viruses. The herpes family includes at least fifty related viruses. Some of these are herpes simplex (the virus that causes cold sores and genital infections), varicella-zoster (the responsible vector for chicken pox and shingles), and Epstein-Barr virus (the causative agent for infectious mononucleosis). There is no reason for terror to strike in your heart when you are informed that your skin problem may be a herpes infection. In the following section, you will see that these viruses affect all of us, that they usually do not produce serious diseases, and that there are good treatments available.

HERPES SIMPLEX INFECTIONS

There are two types of herpes simplex virus (HSV): Type 1 and Type 2. Most people encounter Type 1 virus in the first decade of life. There is usually an asymptomatic infection. However, the virus remains hidden in the nervous system, and years later, for no apparent reason, the virus moves down the nerves and causes a skin infection. Most of these are known as cold sores. These are so-named because they often flare when your resistance is lowered by a cold or the flu.

The first symptoms of an HSV infection are itching, burning, and tingling followed within hours by a red sore that develops small, grouped blisters on a red base. The blisters break, and a scab forms on the surface. The lesion usually heals without a trace within ten days. The most common site of this outbreak is around the lips, although any skin site is possible. Once you have your first outbreak, there is a good chance that you will have additional episodes, usually in exactly the same location. Some people will have one episode every few years, and others will have one sore heal and promptly get a new one.

Most recurrent episodes come and go mysteriously; however, in many instances, sun exposure, a recent illness, or the onset of menstruation can trigger an infection. The natural course of HSV infections of this type is completely unpredictable.

Most genital herpes infections are caused by Type 2 HSV, although some are associated with Type 1 HSV. In most instances, the virus is acquired after sexual contact. The epidemic of HSV Type 2 infections has expanded to the point where up to 20% of sexually active adults have evidence of the virus in their system.

Lesions of genital herpes may be found on the vulva, penis, anus, and buttocks. The first episode can be accompanied by fever, muscle aches, and malaise. Recurrent infections usually do not have such systemic signs. Lesions located on the penis or vagina can be very uncomfortable and may interfere with urination and sexual intercourse.

As with cold sores, lesions of genital herpes are preceded by a feeling of burning, tingling, and itching. The lesions start as red bumps that evolve into grouped blisters. At this stage, the lesion is teaming with infective viruses. This is the stage at which it is most contagious. Once the blisters break and a scab forms over the surface, the viruses disappear and the infection can no longer be spread to others.

Many "miracle" cures for herpes simplex infections have come and gone. There is now one outstanding treatment that can improve the quality of life for the person with recurrent disease. Acyclovir works like an antibiotic to inactivate the virus that infects the skin. Once an infection is established, this drug has only modest beneficial effects. However, if you have recurrent disease, daily dosing with acyclovir can prevent or greatly reduce the number of recurrences that you will experience. The pills are taken twice daily. They have essentially no serious side effects except to your wallet—a month's supply costs over one hundred dollars. They are probably safe, even when taken for years at a time. If you stop the medication, the infections will recur promptly in most situations.

There are no set rules as to who is a prime candidate for long-term prophylaxis with acyclovir. If you get one or two infections a year, the cost of medicating yourself continuously to prevent this minor degree of debility seems high. If you are developing one or more infections a month, this treatment is clearly indicated. For those of you in between these two extremes, discuss the situation with your doctor. The two of you together can weigh the benefits against the cost of therapy.

As a good citizen, it is important that you practice responsible public health behavior during outbreaks of herpes, particularly the genital type. If you have an active genital lesion and engage in unprotected sexual intercourse, it is likely that your sexual partner will get the infection if that person has not yet been exposed to the virus. Condoms can prevent spread of herpes only if the lesion is completely covered. If you have a lesion at the base of the penis and this is not covered by a condom, you are not practicing safe sex. If you have a cold sore on the lip with blisters, kissing can rupture them and spread the virus onto your partner's face. When the lesion has scabbed over completely, you may resume your normal activities.

VARICELLA-ZOSTER INFECTIONS

Chicken pox (varicella) is one of the most common childhood infections. Few people reach adulthood without succumbing to this disease. If the infection is acquired later in life, there can be serious consequences. Once you have recovered from varicella, it is highly unlikely that you will ever have that disease again, but the virus stays in your system for life. When this virus decides to come back for an encore, herpes zoster (shingles) results.

The varicella virus is acquired through airborne droplets from another person with the infection who coughs or sneezes the virus into the environment. Ten to twenty-one days after exposure, there is a brief period of fever and malaise followed by waves of blisters arising on a red base. The entire body may be covered. If there is doubt about the diagnosis, look in the scalp. There are usually lesions present there. Most people with varicella feel fine, except for the itch that often accompanies the eruption. All new lesions arrive within three or four days and usually disappear in ten days. The infected person should be isolated until all the lesions have formed crusts. At that stage he is no longer contagious.

In most cases there is no need to treat the infection. Large doses of acyclovir may reduce the number of days of illness minimally, but the cost of treatment does not justify its routine use. People with certain serious underlying diseases who develop varicella may benefit from acyclovir. If there is substantial itching, you can obtain some relief by pouring a cup of corn starch in tepid running bath water and sitting in the tub for twenty to thirty minutes.

Years after you recover from varicella, the virus may be reactivated and emerge as herpes zoster (shingles). You cannot catch shingles from another person. It comes from within. If you have active herpes zoster, it is possible to spread the virus to someone who has not yet had chicken pox. If that person develops an infection it will be typical varicella, not herpes zoster.

The virus resides in the nervous system and affects the cutaneous nerves when it becomes clinically evident. This can be a very painful disease lasting for months or even longer, because the nerves can be damaged and remain sensitive long after the infection has subsided.

Herpes zoster usually has beginning symptoms of pain or itch in a localized portion of the skin that corresponds to the path of a nerve. This might be on one side of the trunk, on one side of the face, or down one arm. Within a few days, red patches emerge that form clusters of blisters. There may be only a few lesions, or the entire segment of the skin may be covered with them. The pain may be out of proportion to what you see on the skin. In most cases, the eruption clears within two to three weeks. In those over the age of fifty, the pain may remain for a long time. This is known as post-herpetic neuralgia.

For those who have extensive involvement, there are two treatment alternatives for herpes zoster. Large doses of acyclovir may reduce the severity of the infection modestly, but will probably have little effect on the postherpetic neuralgia. Another antiviral medication, famciclovir, may also moderate the disease somewhat and may reduce the postherpes pain as well. Most people with uncomplicated disease do not need these drugs. The pain associated with this infection can be treated with acetaminophen. If this is not effective, your doctor may prescribe a short course of a stronger pain reliever.

6

Sports and Pregnancy: Special Skin Problems

This chapter discusses skin problems associated with two situations that cause many skin ailments but are hardly classified as "diseases." These two special circumstances are sports participation and pregnancy. If you enjoy athletics or if you become pregnant, the chances are almost 100% that you will develop some skin condition. Most of these will be minor annoyances that you can handle without the attention of a medical professional. The theme of this chapter is that your skin problems should not prevent you from enjoying the activities that give you pleasure.

Skin Problems in Athletes

There are many skin conditions that are unique to those who participate in athletics. In addition, the sporting milieu is often an ideal setup for environmental damage to the skin, skin infections, and flares of pre-existent skin diseases.

FRICTION BLISTERS

Blisters are the most common sports injury. They occur only at sites where shearing forces can pull the top layer away from the lower skin layers. All of us have had foot and hand blisters because the underlying supporting tissue is anchored to allow the top layer to separate. You don't get friction blisters in the groin, for example, because this type of tissue anchoring is absent.

A hot, humid micro-environment such as that found in sweaty shoes also contributes to blister formation. Certain people are genetically prone to form blisters, even with minimal trauma. In the army, the lesions that these afflicted individuals get are called "march blisters" because of the severe blistering that occurs even after a short march.

Friction blisters are preventable if you follow certain simple precautions:

- If you wear new athletic shoes, remove them after a few minutes of vigorous exercise and look for "hot spots" on the feet. These are the red areas that evolve into blisters if left unattended. Place a piece of moleskin padding, available in the foot-care section of the supermarket or drugstore, on the red areas, and leave it in place for several days, until you have broken in the shoes. If previous experience has shown you where you always develop blisters, place the pads on those sites before wearing the new shoes for the first time.

- Drying foot powders and absorbent socks can help to keep your feet dry. It may look sporty to go without socks, but your feet will not appreciate it. If you sweat profusely into your shoes, change your socks in the middle of exercising if necessary. Some of the worst blistering I have ever seen occurred in long distance runners who wanted to get a few more miles in after their feet became drenched with sweat.

- If a blister develops, you can drain the fluid by perforating the roof with a pin that has been sterilized in boiling water. Do not remove the blister roof. It acts as a biologic dressing and helps to prevent an infection.

- If you develop blisters no matter what type of footwear you use, consult your physician. It is possible that you have a hereditary blistering disorder that requires special attention.

JOGGER'S NIPPLES

When clothing rubs against the nipples, painful erosions can occur. This happens to women who exercise without wearing bras or to men who work out in shirts made of hard fabrics. This is called jogger's nipples because it is common in long distance runners, but it may occur in tennis players, in those who take aerobics exercise classes, and in participants in other sports as well.

You can easily diagnose yourself if you notice that your nipples are sore after a workout. There may be such extensive erosions that you might see blood on your shirt.

The easiest preventive measure for a woman is to wear a bra when exercising. There are many bra manufacturers who promote special bras for use during exercise. These do help prevent jogger's nipples, but any well-fitting bra will prevent this from occurring. Seamless cups may be slightly better since the seams could conceivably be a source of irritation. Men can exercise without a shirt or wear one made of a soft, smooth fiber such as nylon. One problem that many competitive runners have is that they receive souvenir T-shirts from races. Often, the sponsors try to save some money by giving out poor-quality garments. Donate these to charity and save your nipples some wear and tear. If changing T-shirts does not solve the problem, you can tape your nipples or apply petrolatum as a lubricant to reduce the frictional injury.

BLACK HEEL

If you participate in a sport with quick starts and stops, such as basketball or tennis, you might develop an asymptomatic black spot on your heel. This represents a small bleeding point that occurs as the heel slams against the back of the shoe. This is a completely harmless problem, but it can look much like melanoma, which is a significant problem. If you note such a spot on your heel, follow it closely. If it remains unchanged for over two weeks, see your doctor. He will probably pare off the top layer of the skin. If the spot disappears, it is black heel rather than melanoma.

PIEZOGENIC PAPULES

If you have ever noticed that small, flesh-colored bumps appear on the sides of your feet after a long run or after a hard game of tennis, you probably have piezogenic papules. These are little hernias on your feet. Small tears in the fascia below the skin on the sides of the feet allow tissue to herniate, or bulge, into the more superficial part of the subcutaneous space. The pressure on the feet from running brings these out, whereas normally they would not bulge into these gaps. Usually, the lesions cause no discomfort, but the tissue can occasionally get caught and can produce pain.

If you have these papules and never have symptoms, there is no particular reason to treat them. If an occasional painful bump occurs, elevation of the leg will usually reduce it in minutes. If the discomfort interferes with your activities, you can purchase a heel cup to place into your shoe. This acts like the old fashioned truss by keeping the herniated tissue from extruding. These heel cups can be custom made by a podiatrist or can be bought in the drugstore.

TENNIS TOE

Most of us would prefer to wear comfortable, loose-fitting shoes when we are at play. Unfortunately, when you propel yourself forward in running sports such as tennis or jogging, the foot can push forward and pound against the front of the shoe. This may cause bleeding under the nail plate of the big toe and other toes which stick out from the rest of the foot. This usually produces little or no discomfort, but the blue-black discoloration under the nail remains until the nail grows out.

Tennis toe can be avoided by wearing shoes that hold the foot firmly in place. Certain athletic shoes have adjustable horizontal straps on the outside, which can cinch the foot in place. This may not be particularly stylish, but it is effective.

Some people have difficulty avoiding this problem, regardless of the type of shoe that they wear. This is particularly true of those with a foot anomaly (Morton's anomaly) where the second toe protrudes farther than the big toe. If you have this anomaly, your toe can be protected by a padded sleeve that slips over it. These can be purchased in the drugstore in long strips that can be cut to fit your toes.

INGROWN TOENAIL

Many of us with oversized feet would love to be reincarnated with small, dainty ones. Since you can't shrink your feet, it may be tempting to stuff them into smaller shoes. This may look good, but there is a price to pay for such vanity. When the toes are squeezed together, the nail plate may grow into the fold on the side of the nail; this causes pain, inflammation, and sometimes, secondary infection. These are the signs and symptoms of an ingrown toenail.

The commonsense solution to ingrown toenails is to come out of the closet with your wide feet and abandon the quest for the narrow-foot look. This poses some problem with athletic shoes since there is less selection in the wider widths. A few shoe manufacturers such as New Balance do produce shoes in wide styles. These wider shoes may prevent major discomfort later if you use them before the problem emerges.

If you do develop an ingrown toenail, it is important to rest your foot for several days. All the treatment in the world is doomed to fail if the stimulus that started the process going continues unabated. For those of you who cannot survive psychologically without your daily exercise, this rest period is your opportunity to try another type of aerobic workout that does not require the continual pounding of your feet on the pavement. Two good choices for those recuperating from ingrown toenails are bicycling and swimming.

If the ingrown nail is exuding pus, or if the redness and tenderness do not subside in a few days, you should consult your doctor. You may need antibiotics if there is an infection. In extreme cases, the doctor may suggest that the ingrown portion of your nail be removed surgically. This will put you out of action for at least a week.

Once the inflammation has subsided, you can minimize the chances of a recurrence by keeping the nails trimmed short and by making sure that the edge of the nail does not push into the nail groove. Keeping that corner filed smooth helps. You may also place a wisp of cotton under the nail plate, to guide it over the groove rather than into it. This is a significant hassle when you are eager to get on your way to the tennis court and start showing the world that you haven't slowed down as much as everybody thinks. It is a lot easier to wear correct-fitting shoes in the first place.

GREEN HAIR

If you still have the illusion that blondes have more fun, spend some time at a swimming pool and observe the hair color of the cute little blond children. There is often a greenish tint, which may look good to the MTV generation, but is a nasty surprise to most people who have tried to remove the color from their hair. Chlorine has been wrongly implicated in this problem. The color is actually from copper that is leached from the pool pipes or is a byproduct of copper-containing algaecides. This element fixes to everybody's hair, but the distinctive green hue can be seen only in those with yellow or white locks.

Once this color is firmly established in the hair shaft, it is extremely difficult to remove, so it is important that one shampoo the hair immediately after swimming. Specially formulated shampoos, such as Ultra Swim, contain compounds that can remove the copper and work well at dislodging it before it is permanently fixed.

STRETCH MARKS (STRIAE)

Although stretch marks occur commonly during adolescence, regardless of one's activities, they are one of the occupational hazards of body builders. After repeated mechanical stresses on the skin, the elastic fibers break. This leads to red, depressed lines, which are permanent. Many different approaches have been advocated for improving stretch marks, including vitamin E (which has no beneficial effect on any skin problem), aloe vera, and Retin-A. Nothing works to repair this damage. Spend your money on protein milkshakes instead. They don't do anything beneficial either, but at least they taste good.

If one of your family members suddenly develops striae, severe acne, and a receding hairline, it is possible that he is taking anabolic steroids. These are bad for his health. Don't let this person get away with this irresponsible behavior just to add bulk to his frame.

INTERTRIGO

When you exert yourself, your skin gets warm and moist as you sweat. This is magnified in areas that are normally damp, such as the areas between the toes, in the groin, and in the underarm area. These are excellent breeding grounds for bacteria and fungi. Irritation also occurs as skin rubs against skin in these body folds. This combination of factors leads to intertrigo, which is the combination of inflammation and infection that appears in the right microenvironment. For example, what is called athlete's feet is often a mixed bacterial and fungal infection in the toe web spaces. Treating only one component of this problem is often not successful.

Control of this condition requires that the areas be kept clean and dry. This is a challenge for the athlete who sweats for hours at a time and changes his socks weekly. If you wish to rid yourself of the irritation of an intertrigo, it is important that you pay attention to routine hygiene in these sites. Here are a few simple measures that will improve this condition:

- Apply drying powders before and after exercising.

- Change your socks regularly and bring an extra pair to use for the second half of your workout.

- Dry the affected areas well after showering. For hard-to-get-to areas like the toe web spaces, use a hair dryer at the medium setting to evaporate excess moisture.

If the irritation persists, consult your doctor. He may prescribe creams containing antifungal antibiotics, corticosteroids, or a combination of the two. Request that he give you nothing stronger than hydrocortisone for use in the groin or under the arms. Prolonged use of more potent agents can lead to skin thinning.

EXTERNAL EAR INFLAMMATION AND INFECTION

The ear canal is another warm, moist spot where inflammation and infection commonly occur. This is a particular problem in swimmers whose ear canals stay damp for hours at a time. The cardinal sign of external ear inflammation and infection (otitis externa) is a foul-smelling drainage from the ear canal. This is accompanied by pain, especially if you pull down on the ear lobe.

If you develop this condition, it can only heal if you stay out of the water for at least one week. This can wreak havoc during a competitive swim season; however, halfway measures such as ear plugs and antibiotic lotions will not clear this problem if the ear canals remain wet.

One way of drying out the canals and treating any infection at the same time is to use vinegar soaks. You can use an eyedropper to drip the liquid into the canal, or you can soak a washcloth, apply it to the entrance to the ear canal, and let the excess vinegar drip in. A common practice is to place medicines into the ear canal with a cotton swab. This can damage the mucosal surface and add to your problems, however. There is an old dictum that applies in this situation: Don't place anything smaller than your elbow in the ear canal.

HERPES INFECTIONS

As noted in chapter 5, herpes infections are caused by a virus that resides in the peripheral nerves and travels to the skin to produce clinical disease. When blisters are present, it is a contagious disease. It is easy to spread this virus from person to person during contact sports such as wrestling. Whole teams have been afflicted at the same time and have passed the infection to other teams. There have even been mini-epidemics affecting an entire league. This public-health nightmare is almost completely preventable. If you are a participant in a contact sport and develop a cold sore, you must refrain from practice or from matches until the blisters have crusted over completely. If you are a coach, you must not make exceptions for the star of the team or for a crucial match. It is not worth a lifetime of recurrent infections to the person who catches the viral disease from one of your athletes.

As noted in chapter 5, if you are an athlete who develops numerous herpes infection recurrences, acyclovir therapy will greatly reduce the number of infections as long as you take the medication. You might consider using this drug during the season to protect yourself and others from this annoying skin problem.

CONTACT DERMATITIS

Many sports place the skin in contact with a variety of potential irritants and allergens. For example, if you in-line roller skate, you wear pads containing rubber, and a chin strap made of leather. As you sweat while skating, these materials can be leached from the equipment and onto your skin. If you are allergic to either of these substances, you may develop a contact dermatitis. (See chapter 5.) Those who are wrapped in protective bandages, to protect a sore ankle for example, often apply a sticky substance called benzoin to the dressings to make them adhere better. This is a fairly common allergen.

Contact dermatitis is not hard to spot if you remember that the rash will occur mostly in the areas in direct contact with the offending agent. So if you wear knee pads, the eruption will be over the knees. There will usually be intense itching, accompanied by weeping, oozing, redness, and scaling.

Contact dermatitis is treated with topical corticosteroids. You might try over-the-counter hydrocortisone, but it often is not potent enough to give you major relief of the symptoms. As noted in chapter 5, your physician has many stronger preparations that work better in contact dermatitis.

Once you develop an allergy to a constituent of your sports equipment, every time you wear it your eruption is likely to return. Sometimes, different brands of the same item contain slightly different materials, and one brand may lack the substance you are allergic to. Unfortunately, in many instances, common sensitizers are the culprits. If you love the feeling that you get from in-line skating and wish to continue this form of exercise, there is one trick that may work. If the offending substance can be kept from touching the skin, the rash can be prevented. Try wearing an item of clothing under the padding. This will absorb the sweat that otherwise would extract the offending material from the pad, and it may physically block it from touching the skin. Another way that this can be accomplished is by wrapping a cotton handkerchief around the pad before wearing it.

SUN-INDUCED SKIN INJURY

As I discussed in chapter 4, the sun is not your friend. I strongly recommend that you avoid it if possible. Obviously, many sports are played in the bright sunshine; this is part of the enjoyment of these activities. When you are outdoors for hours at a time, there are a few protective measures that you can take to minimize the damage from the sun without interfering with your fun:

- Try to exercise outdoors before 10 A.M. or after 3 P.M., if possible, because the sun's rays are less intense during these times of day.

- Wear clothing, hats, and sunglasses that cover as much of the skin as is practical. For example, if you swim, wear a cotton T-shirt over your bathing suit. There is not a single sport (except maybe nude volleyball) that absolutely must be played without a shirt.

• As noted in chapter 4, sunscreens are an integral part of any sun protection program. The main problem that sports participants have with these products is that perspiration causes them to run into the eyes, and this burns. Many potent sunscreens are now waterproof; they resist water for hours. Choose one of these products. Sunscreens take a while to absorb into the skin. Remember to apply sunscreen *before* going outside. If you apply it and immediately jump into the pool, you may get a sunburn because the sunscreen did not have a chance to fix itself to the deeper layers of the epidermis. Even waterproof sunscreens should be reapplied after you have been in the water for a while or if you are sweating profusely.

DRY SKIN

One of the most common dermatologic complaints in athletes who are outdoors in the winter is pruritus (itch). Typically, the itching begins just as you have completed a warm-up. If you are a long distance runner, the itch will begin after you have run a couple of miles. By far, the most common cause of itching in this situation is dry skin (xerosis). Forget changing your diet, your laundry detergent, your clothing, or your personal trainer. Instead, lubricate your skin before exercising and after showering. Your itch problem will vanish. (For a complete discussion of moisturizing the skin, see chapter 3.)

PRE-EXISTING SKIN DISEASES

Most people with skin conditions can enjoy the sporting life without any consideration to the adverse consequences of participation. However, there are some skin diseases that can flare with sports activities. This is important for the person who is already involved with sports and for the parents of young children whose athletic interests are just being molded. Both of these issues are addressed in this section.

   Acne mechanica. Many teen athletes will complain that their acne flares during the season. This is particularly true in those playing sports where there is frictional trauma to the acne-prone skin sites such as the chin and upper shoulders. For example, a football player wears a chin strap and shoulder pads. Both of these pieces of equipment rub on the skin and exacerbate pre-existent acne. This is called acne mechanica because mechanical trauma to the skin brings on the flare of the disease. In almost all cases, a person already has acne that is worsened by the sports equipment. Very seldom does someone without a history of acne suddenly develop it during football season. The simplest way to minimize this problem is to wear a shirt under the pads or whatever is rubbing the skin.

Another approach is to use a more aggressive therapeutic regimen during the sports season. Unfortunately, this is not always successful, and the acne may not improve until the season ends. As described in chapter 5, Accutane is an extremely effective acne therapy that often works when all else fails. In cases where there is imminent scarring, this may be very beneficial. There is one problem with Accutane use in athletes. About 15% of Accutane users will have muscle aches, often in the lower back and shoulders. This can affect athletic performance. So think twice before using it if you are a competitive athlete.

Atopic dermatitis. Many children and young adults are troubled by this itchy skin condition. (For a complete discussion, see chapter 5.) Many factors contribute to the itching, or pruritus, that can make the lives of these young people quite unpleasant. Heavy or restricting sports equipment can make them itch. Excess dryness from frequent showering or bathing, which is usually necessary after practices or games, also increases the chances for uncontrollable pruritus.

Many children are diagnosed with atopic dermatitis early in life, before they have developed interests in specific sports activities. If you have an atopic child, consider directing him to sports that won't make his skin disease flare. Sports such as tennis, swimming, soccer, and gymnastics do not require restrictive clothing or padding. Football and hockey would not be good choices.

If your child's skin disease does flare during the season, an aggressive program of lubrication and topical corticosteroids might get him through reasonably well. A few people with recalcitrant atopic dermatitis are on systemic corticosteroids, such as prednisone, for months or even years at a time. These children should avoid contact sports because minor injuries might heal slowly due to the corticosteroids.

Cholinergic urticaria. This is a form of hives that occurs in predisposed people after exertion, sweating, or hot showers. Since these are the very conditions that almost all athletic activities entail, it is not surprising that these individuals have problems when they exercise. They develop minute itchy red bumps which last up to an hour before fading without a trace.

Most people with cholinergic urticaria view it as a minor annoyance. For those whose pruritus is more bothersome, antihistamines can give partial relief. Many athletes, however, do not appreciate the sedating side effects of most of these agents that can affect performance. There is little point in treating this condition after a workout since the treatment does nothing to hasten the disappearance of the lesions, which resolve quickly anyway.

Exercise-induced anaphylaxis. This is an unusual but potentially devastating skin problem that may occur in well-conditioned athletes. While exercising, these people suddenly develop generalized itching, followed by hives, a flushed sensation, a pounding headache, and difficulty in breathing. This is associated with a profound drop in blood pressure, which can lead to shock. (This is the only situation that I can think of where couch potatoes may have reason to gloat.) Once someone has one episode of this form of anaphylaxis, it is likely that he will have additional ones, always without any warning.

The exact cause of this problem is not known. The syndrome is brought on by exercise, but exactly what role exertion plays is not clear. Some people report that certain foods eaten just before exercise bring on an attack, but most do not have this experience.

Once your doctor has made the diagnosis of exercise-induced anaphylaxis, you must change the way you exercise forever. If possible, never exercise alone, especially if you swim or run on deserted roads. Epinephrine is a drug included in insect sting emergency kits. You can save your life by giving yourself an injection of this medication at the first sign of an impending attack. Keep it handy in a backpack near where you are exercising.

There is no foolproof way to prevent these attacks. Antihistamines can help if taken before exercising but are useless after you develop full-blown anaphylaxis. As mentioned earlier, these drugs can detract from your performance. You need to decide whether it is worth it to take a medication chronically to prevent something that may seldom occur.

Skin Changes in Pregnancy

There are many physiologic changes that are associated with pregnancy. As your body alters itself to accommodate to the needs of the unborn child. Your skin is affected even though it's an innocent bystander. There certainly are no important functions that it serves during this period. Most of these skin alterations are of hormonal origin. In this section I describe common findings during pregnancy and abnormal skin conditions that may complicate an otherwise uneventful nine months.

CHANGES IN PIGMENTATION

Up to 90% of pregnant women will develop an increase in pigmentation (hyperpigmentation). It is usually mild and generalized but is particularly evident in areas that normally have more pigment, such as the nipples, the skin around the genitals and anus, and under the arms. In addition, many women develop a dark line called a linea nigra running from the belly button to the area above the pubic hair. This is most pronounced in those with dark complexions. Moles and freckles often darken, as do old scars. This increase in pigmentation begins early in pregnancy and progresses until delivery. The color always lightens after the baby is born, but it may not come back to exactly the same shade as before.

Many women have increased skin color over the cheeks, upper lip, forehead, and chin. The medical term for this entity is melasma (chloasma), but a more descriptive term is "the mask of pregnancy" because the distribution is in the shape of a party mask. It is much more frequent in those with dark hair and dark skin color. It also appears in women on oral contraceptives. Melasma typically is tan to blue-gray and has a lacy, reticulated appearance. In many instances, this color fades after pregnancy, but some women are troubled with it for months or years afterward.

Although there is no way to prevent melasma from occurring, sun protection will help minimize the problem. It is very important that you wear sunscreen when outdoors. The chemicals in these products will not get absorbed into your system, and will have no adverse effect on the baby.

If melasma persists after delivery, your physician can treat you with several different agents that may fade the skin. The most commonly used compound is hydroquinone, which is found in many fade creams. The concentration in these over-the-counter products is low and often insufficient to take care of the problem. Prescription-strength agents work better, but they take months to achieve satisfactory results. Since sunlight will darken the areas that you are trying to fade, sunscreens are essential. One product, Solaquin Forte, contains both hydroquinone and a sunscreen and is a convenient way to treat this condition. In cases where hydroquinone alone does not work well enough, your physician may add Retin-A to the regimen. It appears to have a moderate depigmenting action itself and makes hydroquinone work more effectively.

In intractable cases of melasma, your doctor may recommend a chemical peel. (See chapter 8 for a complete discussion of this procedure.) This is an effective means of removing the unwanted pigment, but there is some risk of an uneven result.

During pregnancy, physiologic changes occur in liver function that lead to an impaired clearance of bile. If this is exaggerated, the bile can back up into the skin, which can turn a yellowish color called jaundice. In almost all women with this problem, there is no important medical consequence to being jaundiced, other than a somewhat sallow, sickly appearance. There is no treatment necessary for this condition; it always resolves after delivery. If, however, there are symptoms such as nausea, vomiting, fatigue, and poor appetite associated with the skin yellowing, your doctor may do some tests to rule out viral hepatitis.

VASCULAR CHANGES
Estrogen levels, which cause the blood vessels to dilate, increase greatly during pregnancy. The effects take many forms; for example, over half of pregnant women have red palms. This may appear as either a diffuse red color or a spotty increase in redness on the heels of the palms. In either situation, this is an entirely innocuous condition that resolves within a few days of delivery.

Small spiderlike red spots, aptly called spider angiomas, first appear between the second and fifth month of pregnancy. They are most notable on the upper chest wall, neck, throat, and face. They consist of tiny red dots with spindly, radiating branches.

Spider angiomas are only a cosmetic concern, and there is no compelling reason to treat them during pregnancy since most will regress after delivery. If they do persist, electrocautery of the central feeder vessel will lead to complete disappearance of the lesions. There may be a scar after this procedure, however.

Varicose veins appear in about 40% of all pregnant women. These can be on the legs or in the rectum (better known as hemorrhoids). The tendency to develop leg varicosities runs in families, so check your mother's legs before you become pregnant to find out what is in store for you.

Varicose veins are widely distended vessels caused by increased intravascular pressure. This occurs because the enlarging uterus pushes on the pelvic veins and prevents blood from returning from the legs. In those who develop this problem, there is some inherent vascular weakness, because there is often evidence of varicosities before the womb has enlarged enough to cause much trouble. Other factors such as prolonged sitting with the legs in a dependent position, standing, and wearing constrictive girdles may also contribute to the severity of varicose veins.

If you are prone to varicose veins of the legs, there are some things that you can do to minimize the problem:

- Watch your weight. The less the pressure from excess pounds that your veins must support, the more likely it is that they won't enlarge.

- Elevate your legs. Try to keep the legs above the level of your heart for at least thirty minutes twice daily. If it is tolerable, put pillows under your legs when you sleep at night.

- Avoid standing for prolonged periods in one position. Sitting with your legs dangling is also not good for varicose veins. Set aside at least twenty minutes each day to walk or swim. These activities allow your muscles to assist the veins in moving blood out of the legs.

- Elastic support hose help a little but are not a substitute for the strategies mentioned above.

If you develop hemorrhoids while pregnant, there are several things that you can do to improve the situation. Sitz baths are soothing and can shrink the swollen tissues. Stool softeners will allow you to strain less when you have a bowel movement, taking some of the pressure off the veins in the rectum. If it takes you more than one minute to complete a bowel movement, you need a stool softener such as those containing psyllium. These work by adding bulk and water to your stool; this stimulates the rectum to discharge its contents.

Bruising of the legs happens quite frequently in the latter stages of pregnancy. It appears as either irregular purple patches or as small purple dots (petechiae). As the pressure builds up in the leg veins, small amounts of blood leak out into the skin, giving it a bruised appearance. If bruising occurs without trauma in other parts of the skin, consult your doctor; there are other blood diseases that could be responsible.

STRETCH MARKS

These are one of nature's cruel little tricks. Stretch marks, or striae, appear during the sixth and seventh months of pregnancy. There appears to be an inherited tendency to develop stretch marks, so if your sister has them you are likely to have them also. Caucasians have more of them than African Americans or Asians. Striae appear as irregular, linear, depressed, pink-to-purple stripes; they are most common on the abdomen, breasts, upper arms, and buttocks.

The prevailing view of the origin of stretch marks is that as you gain weight during pregnancy, the skin stretches to the point where elastic fibers rupture, but it may not be that simple. Hormones secreted from the pituitary gland in large amounts during pregnancy may change the structure of the connective tissue, leading to breakage of the fibers. Stretch marks usually fade over several months after delivery. There is no effective treatment for this problem.

GLANDULAR ACTIVITY

Pregnant women often complain that they sweat more than before they became pregnant. Although the cause is unclear, there is an increase in sweat gland activity. Some think that increased girth may be the reason this happens. It may also have something to do with a change in thyroid gland function. For whatever reason, the pregnant woman's thermostat is set downward; she sweats even when she doesn't feel particularly hot. There is not much that can be done about this situation other than trying to stay as cool as possible in loose-fitting clothing and an air conditioned environment.

Sebaceous glands also increase their activity. This leads to increased oiliness, particularly on the face and upper trunk. Some pregnant women have terrible acne flares, and, presumably, this increased sebaceous activity is responsible. (For treatment tips, see chapter 5.) Remember that when you medicate yourself, the drug is being shared by the developing fetus. Think twice before using systemic medications during pregnancy.

SKIN EDEMA

Swelling of the face, hands, ankles, and feet is a common occurrence during the later stages of pregnancy. It is usually more pronounced in the morning and improves as the day progresses. This edema appears because of sodium and water retention and can be especially severe in those with pre-existent heart or kidney diseases. Toxemia of pregnancy is also associated with generalized edema.

For those with troubling edema, salt restriction can be helpful. An exercise program can reduce leg edema somewhat. Diuretics should be reserved for only the most disabling situations. Take heart; the swelling will disappear soon after delivery of the baby.

ITCH OF PREGNANCY

Itchy skin is one of the most common symptoms near the end of pregnancy. This may be localized, often on the abdominal wall, or may be over most of the skin surface. In most instances, the exact cause is never found. Some unknown factors are finding their way to the skin. At one time, it was thought that liver problems were responsible for many of these cases but this notion has not been proven. Without other signs of liver dysfunction, there is no need to worry about some hidden liver problem if you itch while pregnant.

Pregnant women can acquire itchy (pruritic) skin conditions just like those who are not pregnant. As outlined in chapter 5, underlying dermatoses such as dry skin, scabies, and atopic dermatitis may be responsible. Certain medications can cause itching. Occasionally, internal diseases can also cause pruritus. Urticaria (hives) is frequent during pregnancy, especially in the last two to three months. In most cases, this itchy condition mysteriously appears and just as mysteriously vanishes shortly after the pregnancy is finished.

Treatment of the pruritus of pregnancy is complicated somewhat by the fact that you should avoid internal therapies if possible during pregnancy. Antihistamines such as diphenhydramine and chlorphenaramine are safe for pregnant women, but they don't help the itch of pregnancy much unless it is caused by hives. They will allow you a decent night's sleep if the itch is keeping you awake.

Topical anti-itch remedies do not work well in this situation. Exceptions are oatmeal or corn starch baths, which are soothing and moderately helpful for the temporary relief of symptoms. Another topical therapy that may improve the itch is the ultraviolet light from sunshine exposure. Here is one of the few times when dermatologists will encourage you to sun yourself. Tanning booths are useless in this situation, and topical corticosteroids such as hydrocortisone do not work in the pruritus of pregnancy.

HAIR CHANGES

Most pregnant women will notice at least a mild degree of increased hair growth. This is usually in the areas that men normally have hair, such as the upper lip, chin, and cheeks. It may also be on the forearms, legs, and back. This is more pronounced in those who are more hirsute from the start. If this happens to you, you are not destined to have this problem for life. It usually reverts to the prepregnancy state after delivery. If you become pregnant again, expect to see the hair return to the degree that you had in previous pregnancies.

Many pregnant women report that the hair on the scalp becomes lush during the pregnancy. If this happens to you, enjoy it while you can because it definitely won't last. As noted in chapter 2, the hair goes through cycles of growth, resting, and shedding. During the nine months of pregnancy, more hairs remain in the growth phase. Within a few months of delivery, these hairs cycle into the resting phase and subsequently fall out as new hairs take their place. There are few more panicked people in this world than those who struggle to lose all the weight that they gained while pregnant only to be greeted by massive hair loss a few months later. Expect to lose some hair after delivery. In some instances, up to half of your scalp hair may fall out over a two-to-three month period. You may even need a wig for a few months. Try not to worry. In almost all women the hair eventually begins to cycle normally and they get their old hair density back. It might take up to fifteen months after the start of the hair fall, but it will happen.

NAIL CHANGES

Nails and hair are intimately related structurally and have similar growth properties. Unlike hair, the nails do not have accelerated growth during pregnancy. In some respects, the opposite is the case. They may become soft, brittle, and ridged. They may also separate from the underlying nail bed. These changes are completely reversible; however, since the nails grow slowly, it may be six to nine months before you see absolutely normal nails again. In chapter 7, I outline things to do to improve the appearance of abnormal nails.

7

Cosmetics and Other Over-the-Counter Products

All of us have been endowed with characteristic features that distinguish us from others. Included in our unique attributes are irregular contours, colors, and blemishes that detract from what the world considers a "perfect look." To create the illusion of perfect skin, thousands of different cosmetics have been developed. In many ways, these do an outstanding job of masking minor flaws and improving appearance. There is enough variety from which to choose that almost any person can find some product to suit his or her needs. But it is important to remember that, by definition, cosmetics have no effects on the skin *per se*. They only improve the appearance rather than the structure or function of the skin. This chapter will review cosmetics by the type of agent and the area of the skin where they are used. The main theme will be to choose the look that is right for you (not for a super model who has had extensive plastic surgery) and the products that work best for your unique skin. Much of the information in this chapter was extracted from a book written for dermatologists by Zoe Draelos (*Cosmetics in Dermatology*, Churchill Livingstone, Inc.). It is easily readable by those who are not physicians. If you want details on the subjects covered in this chapter, you should read her book.

Before embarking on the task of picking cosmetics, it is important to determine if you have dry, oily, or a combination of dry and oily skin. A simple test can help you to make this determination. Before washing your face, place a piece of absorbent towel against your skin.

If an oil stain appears at several different sites on your face, you would be classified as having an oily complexion. If few or no sites produce an oil stain, you have dry skin. The presence of scale is not necessary for one to be classified as having dry skin. Most people have combination skin. Some areas are oily and others are not because the concentration of sebaceous glands differs from location to location. Most individuals have more oil glands over the central portion of the face and are oilier there. The sides of the forehead and the portion of the cheeks near the hairline tend to be drier. Remember, surface oils are good for your skin. Those of you with oily complexions are being better protected from drying by these sebaceous gland secretions. Fortunately, there are outstanding cosmetics for every type of skin imaginable, but it is important to get the right match for your skin.

Possible reactions to cosmetics occupy the attention of cosmetic manufacturers and consumers alike. We dermatologists treat many patients with facial eruptions that they ascribe to a reaction to a cosmetic. In fact, only a few of all such rashes that I treat are related to the cosmetics that the patient is using. For the most part, these products are very safe. What a patient may think is an allergy to eye makeup is often seborrhea of the eyelids. Dry skin of the face is often blamed on cosmetics. Even generalized skin eruptions are blamed on products applied to a small area of the skin. Here are some general guidelines to consider before attributing a skin problem to a cosmetic:

- Allergic reactions occur at the site of application of the allergen. If you apply an eyeliner you are allergic to, your eyelid skin should be most prominently involved in any rash although the skin next to it could also react. Don't blame your nail polish if you develop a skin eruption on the hands and feet.

- If you develop a rash immediately after applying something to your skin, it is not an allergic reaction. Allergies take about two days to manifest themselves after contact with the offending agent.

- It is possible to develop an allergy to a cosmetic after years of using it uneventfully. Sometimes these agents are mild allergens and your body takes time to elaborate an immune reaction against them. However, look to the most recently started product as the offender if you get a new eruption.

- With the rare exception of inhaled fumes from cosmetics, there is essentially no danger of having a systemic reaction from the application of these agents to the skin. I am skeptical of claims that chemicals in cosmetics cause chronic fatigue, arthritis, and other ailments.

• Irritant reactions are different from allergies. Theoretically, any of us could develop an irritation from a given cosmetic if we applied enough of it to sensitive skin. This is in contrast to allergic reactions, when only a few of us would have an immune reaction against the chemical. As you might have guessed, irritant reactions are far more common than allergies. If you do develop an irritation from a preparation, it does not necessarily mean that you can never use that particular product again. Smaller amounts, less frequent application, or accompanying moisturizers are often enough to prevent the irritant response.

• If you do suspect an allergy, the most likely culprits are the fragrances or preservatives in a product. If you have a problem sorting this out, your dermatologist can do allergic patch tests to determine what substance you are allergic to.

Facial Cosmetics

The most important component of most makeup programs is the foundation. It is designed to provide even color, cover imperfections, and blend into the uncovered skin. Four types of formulations are available, each of which exploits your skin type to maximize results.

The color of almost all foundations is based on titanium dioxide. If the product has more of this compound, the pigment will be denser. In the past, increased amounts of titanium also meant that the product would feel heavy. Now with a better, micronized form of titanium, you can get good coverage without looking as if you just finished a dress rehearsal for a stage play. Another added benefit is that it is a good sun blocker. By wearing foundations with large amounts of micronized titanium, you are protecting your skin from ultraviolet light to the point where you almost certainly won't burn in the sun, and you may get some anti-aging and skin cancer protection as well. This is further discussed in chapter 4.

If you purchase makeup at a store that does not have salespeople knowledgeable about the products, you might have to do a little experimentation on your own to find out how oily a given foundation is. The names and descriptions of the products often give you no clue about their chemical nature. Exactly how oily is a product called Sheer Beauty? I have no idea, and many marketers would prefer to keep you in the dark as well. An easy way to determine the degree of oiliness is to do a test similar to the one that you performed on your face. Place a drop of the product onto a piece of absorbent paper such as a coffee filter. If no ring appears, the product is probably oil-free. If there is a small ring, there is a relatively minor amount of oil present. As the size of the ring increases, the more oil-based the foundation is.

As with foundations, people with special needs must chose and use all facial cosmetics carefully. If you are troubled with acne, for example, powder blushes are usually best, since they absorb oil and improve the coverage of the oil-free foundations that are recommended for you. Loose powders have less oil than pressed compact powders, making them more easily tolerated by people with acne. Avoid cream rouges; they cover better than powders but they are usually too oily. Bronzing gels are a good alternative for adding color to your face without a great deal of oil.

If you are a mature person, dryness and facial wrinkling make cosmetic application more of a challenge. You should avoid powders, since they tend to be drying and cake in the wrinkle lines, accentuating them unnecessarily. Bronzing gels are difficult to use in furrowed skin and are hard to apply correctly anyway. Cream rouges work best for most older people. They color and moisturize at the same time. Concealers can mask undesirable color tones and lubricate as well.

EYES

Your eyes are often the first feature that someone notices. They express emotions, indicate your state of health, and even show how much sleep you had the night before. Eye makeup can change your appearance remarkably. If your eyes are striking, it can set them off from the rest of your face. If they are small, properly placed cosmetics can magically enlarge them. Spend a little time on your eyes; you could substantially enhance your appearance.

Eye shadows offer you an incredible choice of color, texture, finish, and delivery system. Although current trends will play a part in your choice of eye shadow, your individual needs should be the most important determinant of what you use around your eyes. If you have baggy, redundant eyelid skin, there are a couple of types of eye shadow you'll want to avoid. The first is cream eye shadows, which tend to migrate and gather in skin folds. A setting cream can help the staying power of these eye shadows but probably will not solve your problem completely. The other type to avoid is the pearlescent eye shadows that create a rough texture and enhance wrinkles.

Eyeliners are another popular cosmetic used to enhance the appearance of the eyes. Be careful not to apply them to the inner aspect of the eyelid, because the chemicals can be potentially irritating and they can permanently stain the inner lining of the eye. Liquid eyeliners, which can give you a long-lasting look, produce the most cases of irritant dermatitis of all the forms of eyeliner. Avoid this formulation if you are prone to eyelid irritation.

A popular trend in eyeliners is what is euphemistically called permanent eyeliner. This procedure is performed by some of the most fashionable cosmetic surgeons in the country. They hate it when we say this, but permanent eyeliner is nothing more than a tattoo. It is no different than the Bart Simpson image that your rebellious teenager may have on his buttock. Just as with regular tattooing, an electric needle implants particles of varying shades of blue, brown, or black into the eyelid skin; this truly is *permanent*. You had better like the style and color that the "tattoo artist" uses because you are stuck with it. Of course there are lasers that can remove tattoo pigment, but, believe me, it is a lot more difficult to remove this pigment than it is to implant it. (For more on tattoo removal, see chapter 8.)

The most widely used eye cosmetic is mascara, which thickens, darkens, and lengthens the eyelashes. Waterproof mascaras are a popular solution to smudging. These solvent-based mascaras contain no water. This allows them to stay on better, but they must be removed with a cleanser specifically designed for their removal. Be careful when using these removers because they may be eye irritants. A good alternative is a hybrid mascara, which consists of an emulsion of water-based and solvent-based materials. These are more waterproof than water-based products, dry more rapidly, and are easier to remove than solvent-based products.

Some eye cosmetics can get under a contact lens and cause eye irritation. A simple preventive measure is to place the contact lenses in your eyes *before* applying your eye makeup. In this way the lens itself may protect your eye from injury. If you wear soft lenses, water-based mascaras can absorb onto them and produce staining. Try one of the solvent-based products instead.

LIPS

Cosmetic preparations for the lips not only color and accentuate the lips, but many of these products also cover defects, moisturize, and act as a sunscreen. The lips are particularly vulnerable to sun damage because they lack the melanin pigmentation that protects the skin.

Lipstick is the staple of most makeup programs. The big challenge with lipsticks is staying power. Some lipsticks contain stains that remain long after the lipstick has been removed, but problems with bitter taste and allergic contact dermatitis have limited their use. There are a few nonstaining or film-forming lipsticks. These contain a dye that is deposited on the lips. Another variation is frosted lipstick, which contains minute particles that give the lips a shimmering look.

Lip cream is a creamier way to color your lips. It comes out of a jar rather than from a stick. These creams are applied with the fingertip and impart a shine. However, they are oily and tend to run into crevices around the lips. For the person who smokes and has smoker's wrinkles around the mouth, lip creams will probably accentuate those lines as the color migrates into the small furrows. Lip sealants can help color bleeding somewhat. They are applied under the lipstick and allowed to dry before the lipstick is applied.

Lip liners are used by those who want their lips to look more defined. They are similar to lipsticks but are stiffer and can be applied in a fine line with a pencil. Makeup artists have a method for applying lip liner that may work for you. They outline the lips first with a color that matches the lipstick, and then fill the lips in completely with the liner. This trick helps the color stay on longer by staining the lips, but it can also dry them out because the liner is less waxy than lipstick.

For the person with a lip deformity, lip tattooing is a permanent way to change the contour of the lips. Just like permanent eye liners, once you decide to embark on this procedure there is no turning back. Since it is directly related to the skill of the operator, get several recommendations before you choose the person to do this for you. Remember, styles change, including lip configuration. Don't get a permanent revision of your lip margin just because it's in style. Lip liners are a lot simpler to remove than tattoo pigment and can change the shape of your lips almost as well.

There are a few special lip problems that require additional attention to lip cosmetics. Many older individuals have brown spots (lentigines) or blue bumps (venous lakes) that are difficult to mask with ordinary lipsticks. Lipsticks with a high concentration of titanium dioxide cover better than lip creams or lip pencils. Foundation with titanium under your regular lip cosmetic will achieve the same end. Darker red colors also will mask these blemishes.

Nail Cosmetics

We have evolved with fingernails because they give us the ability to grip objects and protect the tips of our fingers from the inevitable trauma associated with using our hands. For cultural reasons the fingernails, and to some extent the toenails, have taken on an importance out of proportion to their functional properties. In some cultures, long fingernails are an indication that a person belongs to the leisure class, one who does not have to stoop to working with his hands. If a person has nails that are six inches or more in length, his hands are rendered useless because of these unwieldy appendages, but he is at the top of the social heap. In our society clean nails are a sign that you are fastidious. The hidden message is not that different from that of the long-nail society: "I don't work with my hands to make a living." Perfectly formed nails may be a condition of your employment. I have had patients who pleaded with me to do something about their diseased nails, because they could not face the world with malformed nails. These people have even had disfiguring skin conditions elsewhere on their bodies, but their nails were still most important. In some societies painting the nails is an accepted part of a makeup regimen. In other cultures only prostitutes color their nails, often with elaborate designs.

The cosmetic industry has supplied us with many ways to make our nails look luxurious. There are also products that can improve the integrity of the nail plates. In the following section, I will discuss several of these agents and describe some of the problems associated with their use.

NAIL POLISH

Few cosmetics enjoy more widespread use than nail polish. They all consist of film formers that resist abrasion and add gloss and stickiness to the preparation. These ingredients are dissolved in a solvent (the part of the product that produces the smell and the vapors as they evaporate). Any color under the sun can be added to this system to give you the exact shade that you desire. Special effects can be achieved by adding various fillers. Chopped aluminum, gold, or silver can impart a metallic shine, and fish scale or ground synthetic pearl can give the nail a frosted appearance.

If you choose to have a professional manicurist polish your nails, the process can get complicated. First, a base coat is applied to help the enamel adhere better to the nail plate. It also protects the nail from being stained by the coloring agent. (Don't worry if your polish stains, it does not penetrate deeply into the nail plate and usually wears off after a couple of weeks.) Next, the colored nail enamel is applied. A clear topcoat is then added over the color. It contains film formers and plastisizers, which impart a sheen to the nails and add some strength and durability to the nail coating.

Nail polish seldom causes problems, even in those who are sensitive to a number of cosmetics. Since the products do not contain water, there is no need to include a preservative to prevent bacterial contamination. Occasionally a person does develop an allergy to one of the ingredients. This is manifested by redness, tenderness, weeping, and oozing from the skin around the nails. Another possible site of the allergic reaction is the eyelids. This happens because the eyelid skin is thin and reacts readily to allergens. If a person is allergic to a nail polish and scratches or rubs her eyelids, a tiny amount of the allergen could get onto the eyelid skin and cause a reaction. Hypoallergenic nail enamels are available for those who have difficulty finding a polish that doesn't inflame the skin. These products contain fewer chemicals, but there is no guarantee that a similar reaction won't occur.

NAIL POLISH REMOVERS

As alluring as a nail polish can look in the bottle, it can surprise you by being too bold, plain, dull, or shiny when it's on your nails. If the polish needs to come off in a hurry, there are several types of remover available. Solvents containing acetone or various alcohols dissolve the enamel almost instantaneously. But these can be drying to the surrounding skin. Some formulations contain conditioning ingredients such as lanolin and synthetic oils that minimize the irritant effects of the main compound. They are worth using. Be careful with any of these products around flames; they are all highly flammable.

CUTICLE REMOVERS

For some reason, the cuticle is seen as an ugly appendage of the nail that should be removed to enhance one's beauty. This is too bad since the agents that are marketed to dissolve excess cuticular tissue are potential irritants. They can cause inflammation of the tissue around the nail, called a paronychia. Bacteria can gain access to the deeper portions of the skin through this inflamed tissue, possibly leading to major problems that could result in a permanent disfigurement of the nail plate. Please take this bit of unfashionable advice: Don't mess with your cuticles and don't let your nail technician manipulate them either.

NAIL HARDENERS

For those with brittle nails that break off so frequently that they never get long, nail hardeners may be helpful. Hardeners have gotten a bad reputation because they formerly contained free formaldehyde, a chemical that can cause allergic contact dermatitis. Nail hardeners sold in the United States no longer contain formaldehyde, although they may be available in other parts of the world. Hardeners function primarily as a base coat to improve adherence of the colored polish. They also give the nail increased strength, although the results are not dramatic. Some specialty products contain additives such as nylon fibers or other proteins, which are meant to reinforce the nail plate.

ARTIFICIAL NAILS

For the woman who is unable to grow the nails she wants, artificial nails are a good substitute. Depending on how much time and money you wish to spend to get great looking nails, there are several choices. Numerous colors, shapes, and sizes are available to match with your existing nail. If these pre-formed nails are not satisfactory, there are also custom-made sculptured nails.

Pre-formed nails (press-on nails) are easy to apply and remove. They are made with cured plastic, which is nonallergenic. However, the adhesive may cause reactions that lead to a separation of your natural nail (onycholysis), inflammation (paronychia), or loss of the cuticle. There are two ways these plastic structures are fixed to the underlying nail. If you react to one adhesive, you will not have better luck with the other method, since the glues are similar in structure. The simplest adhesion technique is with an adhesive already affixed to the underside of the artificial nail. The other method uses an acrylic glue that you paint on and then fix the artificial nail to.

Whichever form of adhesive is used, the nails should be removed after forty-eight hours to give your nails a chance to "breathe." If the nails are allowed to stay in place for an extended time, moisture, dirt, and bacteria can wedge under them and damage your real nails.

Another variation is nail tips, which are artificial nails applied to the ends of your natural nails. These add length to short nails; however, using them is a bit more involved than other types of press-on nails. An acrylic solution is painted over the whole nail surface to even out the irregularities between the artificial and natural structures. If this substance gets onto the cuticle it can lead to irritation and possible infection.

Nail wraps can also be used to give the appearance of a longer nail. The wrapping is made of paper, silk, linen, or another pliable material and is attached to the nail with an acrylic glue or sealer. After it dries, it can be shaped to conform to the shape of a normal nail tip. It can also be covered with colored nail enamel.

If you want the ultimate in artificial nail beauty and are willing to pay big bucks for it, sculptured nails are an excellent alternative. These are custom-made to fit perfectly onto your own nails. The sculptures are made of a methacrylate polymer, which can cause allergic reactions. The length and color are up to you. When done properly, they look almost exactly like regular fingernails.

If these look so spectacular, why shouldn't everyone do this and forget other less effective methods? There are problems associated with sculptured nails. The major one is that only individuals who are experts in this technique can give you the best results. There is no state regulation of this industry, so anyone can put up a sign as a sculptured nail expert. When done in a slipshod fashion with nonsterilized equipment, infections and nail damage can occur.

Another problem with this technique is that once you are with the program, you and your nail technician get to know one another all too well, since the nails need to be filled in about every three weeks. Failure to do so leads to loosening of the sculptures and a steady deterioration in their appearance. It may wind up costing you five hundred dollars or more per year to maintain your artificial nails.

When used for months at a time, the underlying nails can become dry, thin, and discolored. Eventually they may no longer be able to support the nail sculptures. It is for this reason that many experts recommend that they be worn for no more than three months at a time before a one-month rest period.

8

Options in Aesthetic Surgery

Let's face it, you aren't getting any younger. You work out at the gym three times a week, watch your diet, think clean thoughts, and even assist people older than yourself across busy intersections. But you still are aging by the minute. (Eventually, people are going to ask whether *you* need help crossing busy intersections.) You have tried every nostrum in chapter 7. You have even secretly ordered exotic potions, which are delivered through the mail in plain brown wrappers with instructions written in a language that you can neither read nor understand. Is this the end of the road for you as a useful and beautiful member of society? Not necessarily.

Over the past several decades, many excellent surgical procedures have been perfected that can improve your appearance. In most cases there is a stiff price to be paid out of pocket and some short-term unpleasantness, but the results can be quite gratifying. Before detailing the specific procedures, there are some consumer strategies that are generally applicable.

Don't be ashamed to be vain. A common conversation in my office starts out something like this: "I shouldn't be bothering you about such a trivial thing as the wrinkles on my face. I am too old to be this vain." My reply is usually along the lines of: "It's your body and you have every right to want to look as good as you possibly can. You should have absolutely no apologies for these feelings." What concerns me is when people stop caring about how they look.

Men in particular often think that dwelling on their appearance in public is somehow not in keeping with the Marlboro man demeanor. Many of these are the same fellows who spend half the morning blow drying their hair. Nobody would criticize a man for carefully picking the right tie to complement his suit. All of this makes us feel better about ourselves, and there is nothing wrong with that.

Shop before you buy. Cosmetic surgery is a major undertaking, much like remodeling a house. You certainly would not use the Yellow Pages to select a contractor at random to remodel your home. A similar degree of care must be exercised when choosing the doctor to perform your surgery. There are no foolproof means of determining who is the best person for the job, but it is prudent to talk to at least two surgeons before deciding. Many dermatologists, plastic surgeons, and head-and-neck surgeons are capable of performing these types of procedures. It might be worthwhile to discuss your case with physicians in different specialties to get varying perspectives.

If you know satisfied customers, word-of-mouth recommendations are very valuable. If you receive care by a dermatologist, he will probably know who in your community has special expertise in the procedure you wish to have performed

Most surgeons will arrange a pre-operative interview to discuss your needs and expectations and describe the details of the surgical procedure that is being considered. This is the time to ask all your questions and to get a general feeling whether this is the doctor that you want to perform the surgery. As I discuss in chapter 1, there are times when it just doesn't click between a patient and her physician. You must go into this with trust in your doctor. If you have even minor misgivings, postpone your decision until you are completely comfortable with it. Your friend may have had a marvelous experience with a given physician, and you may have absolutely no rapport with him. I am constantly amazed how one patient thinks that I walk on water and the next can't believe that they let me graduate from medical school. Patients tend to gravitate toward physicians who satisfy not only their medical needs but also their issues of comfort, trust, and general demeanor. I have a very unscientific approach for you to try. Determine if the patients in the waiting room with you have attitudes, expectations, and even personality characteristics similar to yours. If these people look, act, and think like you do, you just may have found the right doctor for yourself.

Try to educate yourself about the therapeutic alternatives *before* you make an appointment with the surgeon. I hope after reading this chapter you will be knowledgeable. If you come armed with the facts, you will probably understand the doctor's explanations better, and you will almost certainly be able to contribute to whatever final decisions are made.

The costs of most cosmetic procedures vary wildly, depending on the community, the specialty of the physician, and even the financial resources of the individual patient. Since almost none of this is covered by insurance, be prepared to pay hundreds or even thousands of dollars at the time of service.

As a part of your search for the appropriate physician, costs often are an important factor in a decision. However, this is not like buying a new home where more money usually means more house. There is little or no correlation between physician charges and skill level. As a rule, dermatologic surgeons are less expensive than plastic surgeons or head-and-neck surgeons. Depending on the procedure, dermatologists may be more skilled than the higher priced specialists. An example of this is injecting filling materials for scar revision. In the normal course of practice, dermatologists inject the skin more often than do most plastic surgeons and can usually do it better. On the other hand, plastic surgeons would probably be better suited to perform a face lift than would the vast majority of dermatologic surgeons. Although it will cost more, in this case it would be worth the extra expense.

Have realistic expectations. Modern surgical techniques can go a long way toward improving your appearance, but do not expect to look the same as you did when you were a teenager. You can look better and you may look younger, but it is unlikely that all the change that you would hope for will happen. No thoughtful surgeon will promise this, because it just does not turn out that way.

Before seeing the doctor for your pre-operative consultation, try to set goals that you would like to achieve and then decide approximately what percentage of improvement would be good enough to go ahead with the operation. If a modest change for the better is worth the trouble and the surgeon can predict (note that I did not say "promise") this degree of success, you will be pleased with the results. If, in spite of the surgeon's measured optimism, you insist on or fully expect perfection, you may be one very unhappy person. Remember, just because your friend looks like a million bucks after her facial peel, you are not guaranteed the same result—even if both of you choose the same person to perform the procedure.

Physicians will often present a portfolio of photographs showing a sampling of the procedures that they have performed. You can trust that these are not going to be examples of the procedures that did not come out well. There are times, however, when the doctor may wish to illustrate a potential side effect of a particular operation or show you what you might look like a few days after the operation is performed. If your prospective surgeon does happen to reveal the range of results— from excellent to not-so-good—this may be the physician for you. I say this because it takes a high degree of self-confidence to display the full range of outcomes.

Don't be the first person in town to "benefit" from a new procedure. The newspapers are full of marvelous new medical break- throughs that can change our lives. The reality is that progress comes extremely slowly, and incremental advances are far more common than giant leaps. This is equally true about cosmetic surgery. Some of the most effective surgical means of improving one's appearance have not substantially changed for decades. When in doubt, go with a method that has stood the test of time.

A corollary to this general guideline is that if a technique is brand new, the surgeon is also new at performing it. He might have just learned about it at a recent medical symposium and be eager to get some experience. Somebody has to be the first patient to have a proce- dure done on her. Try to avoid being that person.

Expect to look worse before you look better. I often advise patients that cosmetic surgery is like an investment. You need to undergo the pain of parting with something that you already have to get a chance at something better. With most of the aesthetic surgery procedures described in this chapter, there is a postoperative healing period that can last up to several weeks, during which you may not be presentable.

Try to plan your schedule *before* you see the doctor, so that you can arrange a recuperation period. You may feel fine within a day after one of these operations, but you may not look so great. Don't decide to get a dermabrasion two weeks before your daughter's wedding and expect to get rave reviews for your appearance. Another important rea- son for you to see photographs of other patients taken soon after their surgeries is to gauge how you will look.

Chemical Peeling

Over the past decade, chemical peeling (also called "chemexfoliation" by those trying to impress you) has emerged as one of the most popu- lar and effective means of improving superficial wrinkling, sun dam- age, pigmentary irregularities, and superficial scarring. This is to be differentiated from the superficial exfoliation that occurs with some of the agents discussed in chapter 3. With those products, only the top (horny) layer of the skin is removed, and the beneficial results are minimal and short lived. Real chemical peeling causes sloughing of the epidermis and a portion of the underlying dermis as well. To refresh your memory on the anatomy of the skin, see chapter 2.

Depending on the nature of the problem, there are several different methods of peeling. One of the advantages of having a physician who is experienced in many of these techniques is that you will have a range of options to suit your needs. This is why I would strongly suggest that you avoid having a surgical peel performed by a nonmedical person, such as a cosmetologist, a health club operator, or a beauty consultant. These people do not have the scientific background to make wise choices for you about the best approach for your individual problem. Anyone can apply an acid to your skin. There are many variables that determine the depth and consistency of a chemical peel. These include the sebaceous gland density and activity, the application of peel enhancers (keratolytic agents, etc.), skin preparation and degreasing, the concentration of the agent used, and the actual technique of the application. If it were my face, I would like to have the operator understand the anatomy and physiology of my skin and choose a course of action based on my needs rather than what particular brand of "secret formula" he happens to carry.

The type of agent chosen and the way that it is used determines the depth of peeling. In the following paragraphs, I will discuss the indications for the various types of peels and take you through a typical treatment session. These treatments do have some risks associated with them, and potential pitfalls of the various techniques will also be presented.

Chemical peeling is an art, rather than a cookbook exercise. Your doctor may choose to approach it somewhat differently than the way that will be described here. That does not mean that he is behind the times (or ahead of the times, for that matter). There is no single, foolproof means of achieving the desired result. Beware of the practitioner who touts a magic formula but refuses to divulge its contents. He might have something to hide.

SUPERFICIAL PEEL

Superficial peels are relatively risk free and cause only minimal discomfort to the patient. Several different agents, including trichloroacetic acid (TCA); a combination of resorcinol, salicylic acid, and lactic acid (Jessner's solution); and so-called "fruit acids" (alpha hydroxy acids) such as glycolic acid are used. These are sometimes called "freshening peels" because they cause minor changes that are often just enough to "tune up" your skin.

The main indications for this type of chemical peel are acne with prominent blackheads and whiteheads (comedos), mildly sun-damaged skin with fine wrinkles and keratoses, pigmentary changes from melasma (see chapter 6) or other causes, and shallow scars from old chicken pox, acne, and so forth. If you have deep wrinkles or furrows or deep pitted acne scars, this is not a useful approach for you. The main problem with this form of therapy is that the improvement is temporary, so a program of repeated treatments is necessary to maintain a good initial response. You may need up to twenty treatments per year. Although an individual treatment session is usually reasonably priced, this could get a little expensive

If you choose this mode of therapy, your doctor might want you to pretreat yourself with Retin-A or one of the alpha hydroxy acid preparations for at least one or two weeks. This removes surface scale and allows the peeling agent to penetrate better and more evenly. Be prepared for a *series* of treatments before there is measurable improvement. Undergoing a single peel just before a big date or a vacation will probably do you little good. A common schedule is weekly or twice monthly sessions until maximum improvement is achieved.

If you decide to have a superficial peel, this is what to expect and what you can do to maximize the result:

- It is a good idea not to wear makeup on the day of the treatment and, perhaps, on the day before as well. Don't use moisturizers, cold cream, or greasy sunscreens either. Anything on the skin that prevents an even coating of the acid solution or penetration of the material will detract from the benefit of this procedure.

- You will be asked to lie down on the examination table, and your eyes will be covered with a gauze pad to prevent any of the acid from dripping into your eyes. Your skin is then cleansed with either alcohol or soap and water to remove surface oils, makeup, and dirt. It is then scrubbed with acetone to dry the surface.

- For the first treatment, a single coat of the peeling material is applied with a damp gauze or with cotton swabs. The material is applied in a weaker strength, in case you have an exceptional sensitivity to the acid. If the reaction is tolerable, heavier coats or higher concentrations of the peeling agent will be used in subsequent sessions.

- Expect to have an almost immediate, flushed feeling in the treated skin. This is accompanied by reddening, which usually lasts for a few days. After two or three days, the skin begins to peel, much as a sunburn would. Your skin might look as if you had stayed out in the sun a little too long. It may feel sensitive for up to a week after the treatment. If you have a dark complexion, the skin peeling can appear exaggerated because the flakes are a darker color. One week after the peel, your skin should be almost back to normal and ready for another treatment.

- In many instances, your doctor will adjust the dosage and the intervals between treatments as you progress with the program. As I mentioned earlier, this is not an exact science, and adjustments in midstream are the rule rather than the exception.

- Any skin problem associated with redness will remain red longer if exposed to sunlight. So it is important that you wear highly protective sunscreens during these treatments. Many people plan their peels during the winter months to avoid this pitfall.

- After a maximum benefit is reached, the peels will be discontinued; however, your doctor may ask that you use either Retin-A or one of the alpha hydroxy acids as a part of a maintenance program to keep your skin looking good. This is particularly true if you have acne with many whiteheads or blackheads.

If superficial peeling sounds too good to be true, you are beginning to get the right idea about this procedure. Many doctors swear by this method of skin freshening, but the reality is that the beneficial effects are usually modest. If you are looking for small benefits with little investment in pain and temporary disfigurement, superficial peeling is an option to consider.

MEDIUM-DEPTH PEEL

If you are not satisfied with a little improvement in your skin and are willing to undergo a fair amount of discomfort, you will get a much bigger return for your investment with a medium-depth peel. This procedure causes a slough of the entire epidermis and the superficial part of dermis. It is useful in correcting sun-damaged skin, keratoses, and fine wrinkles that occur after a lifetime of sun exposure. (See chapter 4 for a detailed discussion of what the sun can do to the skin.) This mode of therapy is particularly effective for the fine crow's feet around the eyes. It is only modestly helpful in correcting the deeper furrows that occur around the mouths of smokers. (All those critics were right—smoking is bad for you.) It can also partially correct shallow scars. As you can see, the same kinds of problems are treated with either a superficial or medium-depth peel. Therefore, you and your doctor must decide exactly how profound the damage is and how aggressive you want to get to correct it.

Before you jump on the peel bandwagon, note that there are some circumstances where a peel is not an appropriate therapy. Here is a partial list that outlines what peels *cannot* do:

- Peels cannot change pore size. As described in chapter 2, pores can't open and close and cannot shrink, regardless of what procedure is performed.

- Peels cannot tighten lax skin. If you have the dreaded turkey neck, consult a plastic surgeon about a face lift. Don't waste your time and money on a chemical peel.

- Peels cannot correct deep, pitted scars from old acne, chicken pox, or other trauma. The skin slough does not go deep enough in medium-depth peels to make a meaningful change in these lesions. If you are really bold, consider a deep chemical peel.

- Peels will not completely fade pigmented spots, especially in dark-skinned individuals. This pigment often lies deep in the skin, far below where the peel will have an effect.

- Peels cannot remove broken blood vessels on the face. Certain types of lasers will work on these unsightly lesions, however. (Lasers will be discussed later in this chapter.)

If you and your doctor conclude that a medium-depth peel will be beneficial, here is what to expect from the procedure:

- As with superficial peels, most doctors pretreat patients with Retin-A or an alpha hydroxy acid preparation for at least two weeks before the actual treatment session. You might get a little ahead of the game by starting on one of these preparations while you are considering whether to undergo the procedure.

- On the day you are scheduled for the peel, do not wear any make-up. Anything on the skin surface that blocks the penetration of the acid might cause an uneven effect.

- Once you are placed in the operating suite, you will probably be given a hospital gown to wear and will be asked to lie down on a surgical table. In most instances, you will not be given any sedatives or pain medicines for this type of peel. If you are the anxious type, ask for a mediction to calm you down a bit. This should be discussed with your doctor in advance.

- The procedure itself involves three steps. The first is to cleanse and degrease the skin. This is done by scrubbing with a soap solution followed by acetone. Sometimes, two rounds of this cleaning are necessary to dry the skin.

- The second phase of the procedure is the application either of a combination of weak acids or of solid carbon dioxide. This prepares the skin for the third phase and ultimately allows for a deeper penetration of the stronger acid to follow. You will feel a burning sensation when this is applied, but it is easily tolerable. Your doctor may provide you with a small hand-held fan to help cool your skin.

- The final step is the application of the main peeling agent, which is usually trichloroacetic acid but may be another equally potent chemical. There will be an immediate burning sensation as the peel solution is swabbed on your skin. This subsides after a few minutes and recurs just after the procedure is completed. Your doctor will apply cool compresses that will relieve the discomfort promptly.

By the time you return home, the peeled skin will be very red, somewhat swollen, and scaly. If the areas around the eyes were peeled, there may be enough swelling to close the lids. In other words, don't plan that big date on the night of your facial peel. Over the next few days, the desquamation (shedding) intensifies and the redness increases, but you will have less discomfort day by day. By the end of the first week, your skin will look as if you had a sunburn. This can be covered by cosmetics until it fades after two or three weeks. Your doctor will urge you to avoid excessive sun exposure and wear potent sunscreens for several months after the peel so that the redness fades quickly.

Several problems associated with medium-depth peeling may occur as the healing process takes place, in spite of careful attention to every detail. Sometimes, the redness lasts longer than usual, occasionally for several months. This is partially avoidable by sun protection. If you are prone to dark marks after skin injury, you may wind up with patchy pigment in the areas that were peeled. Your skin may heal with a slightly different texture than before. For example, it may feel bumpier and somewhat more irregular than you might like. Worse yet, actual scarring might occur in the peeled skin. In most cases, none of these things happen, but if you are feeling unlucky or your astrologer advises against even minimally risky endeavors, you probably should not have a chemical peel.

Infections can occur in peeled skin. This is particularly true in people who, for one reason or another, are prone to such problems. For example, if you have a history of viral fever blisters (herpes infection) of the lip, the virus may re-activate after a peel and the infection may spread over much of the face. Thus, to prevent recurrent herpes infections, your doctor may prescribe a drug, acyclovir (Zovirax), to be taken from a few days before the procedure to a few days afterward.

You can realistically expect to see definite improvement in your appearance after a medium-depth peel. Your friends and family will still be able to pick you out in a crowd, but it is possible that people will comment that you look younger and better.

DEEP CHEMICAL PEEL

As you would imagine, a deep chemical peel extends deeper into the skin to more effectively correct deep-seated damage. This form of deep peeling is effective for moderate facial lines, including smoker's furrows around the mouth. If this is so effective, why bother with the more superficial procedures at all? The reason is that there are all kinds of potential problems with this form of therapy. Unless you are either very desperate or very adventurous, you should pass on the deep peel. Relatively few dermatologists use this form of treatment, and the reasons why will become obvious shortly.

Although there are several ways in which this procedure can be accomplished, most use the chemical phenol to produce the desired effect. It is usually performed on fair-skinned individuals only because of the posttreatment pigmentation that occurs more commonly in dark-skinned people. The procedure is often done in an operating room, because the chemical can get absorbed into the circulation and can, rarely, produce heart rhythm problems, and these are better managed in the operating room.

If you and your doctor agree that a deep peel is the procedure of choice, this is what to expect:

- You will be asked to undergo an extensive pre-operative evaluation, which includes a medical history, a physical examination, a laboratory evaluation, and, if you are over forty, an electrocardiogram and a chest X-ray. Your doctor may also include a test for HIV, since there may be some postoperative oozing of blood as the skin sloughs.

- Shortly before the procedure, you will be premedicated with a painkiller and a sedative. These may make you groggy, but you will not be completely asleep.

- Following the degreasing process described earlier, the phenol is applied with a cotton-tipped applicator or a gauze pad. During the application, you will feel a burning sensation in spite of the premedication that you were given. If this discomfort is severe, an anesthesiologist in attendance may give you additional anesthesia.

- After the chemical has absorbed into the skin, some surgeons place a tape wrap, which is almost like a mask, over the treated area and leave it in place for two days. The purpose of the tape is to enhance the penetration of the phenol. If you believe in the "no pain, no gain" rule, you will appreciate the taping maneuver. It adds to the general discomfort of the procedure but might improve the ultimate outcome.

- For several days after the peel, you will have pain, itching, swelling, redness, and oozing of the skin. There will be crusts that you will gently remove with wet soaks. There may be some bleeding as the skin sloughing occurs. Moisturizing creams may ease the dry feeling caused by all the peeling.

- By the tenth postoperative day, almost all the peeling will have ceased, but your face will still be quite red and may stay that way for up to several weeks. There may be some transient blotching, as some areas heal faster than others.

- As with the medium-depth peel, you will be advised to avoid sun exposure for up to three months to prevent prolonged redness.

All the adverse reactions noted for the medium-depth peel apply to the deeper chemical exfoliation. There are also additional problems that may arise. Small inclusion cysts (milia) may appear in the treated area. These can be treated with gentle extraction by your doctor. The skin may become excessively thin, a condition known as skin atrophy. It can contribute to a change in the skin texture after peeling. Scarring also occurs more often with deeper peels than with the more superficial procedures.

After all of this, why would anyone in their right mind ever want to undergo a deep peel? The answer is that the results can be very impressive. You can look years younger after a phenol peel. Is it worth it? It depends on how much you value a more youthful appearance and how much risk and shot-term pain you are willing to endure for a long-term benefit.

Dermabrasion

Your teenage years are far behind you, and the memories of those awkward times have faded, thank goodness. However, there may be one remnant of your past that stares you in the face when you look in the mirror every morning—your acne scars. As discussed earlier, chemical peeling is one method of reducing these scars, but they are often too extensive for peeling to be a reasonable option.

For many years, dermatologic surgeons have been removing skin irregularities with dermabrasion, a procedure that was inspired by the carpenters of the world who smooth rough surfaces with a plane. In the case of dermabrasion, rather than a broad blade, there is a rapidly rotating wheel or circular brush that removes the surface of the skin.

Dermabrasion not only smoothes out scars but can also remove actinic keratoses, fine wrinkles, and tattoos. This is not a procedure for everyone with these problems, however. If you have a dark complexion or are prone to excessive scarring (keloids), the dermabraded areas can wind up looking worse than before. If you have deep-pitted scars, this method is inappropriate because as the planing goes deeper, the more likely it becomes that new, unsightly scars will be produced to replace the old ones.

Before you rush out to change your appearance with dermabrasion, there are a few general facts that you should be aware of:

- This is a real operation, with bleeding and some pain. If you are not willing to endure discomfort and a less-than-optimal appearance for a couple of weeks, don't consider dermabrasion.

- The results are operator dependent. By that I mean that I would not want to be the first person on whom a fledgling dermabrader tried out a new technique that he had just read about in a medical journal. It takes experience and a real touch to do this correctly. A skilled surgeon can virtually sculpt your face so that the specific variations in the surface texture can be evened out. This is a definite advantage over chemical peeling, where there is less control over the ultimate outcome. Get recommendations from your dermatologist and from those who have undergone the procedure. I would not look for a cut-rate deal and skimp on quality. Your face is too important for that approach.

- Even in the best of hands, don't expect perfection. The degree of improvement ranges from about 20% to 75%—it is *never* 100%. As I will explain shortly, you will be substituting one kind of scar for another. The days of your smooth-as-a-baby-bottom face are over. Don't expect the surgeon to turn the clock back that far.

- The procedure can be performed multiple times on the same site. Theoretically, if you are not completely satisfied the first time, you have another opportunity for additional improvement. However, the degree of benefit may diminish considerably with each procedure.

- In almost all cases, insurance companies regard dermabrasion as a purely cosmetic procedure (except, perhaps, when actinic keratoses are treated). This will be expensive, although prices vary greatly between practitioners.

- If you have recently finished a course of Accutane for acne (see chapter 5), you will need to wait at least six months before undergoing a dermabrasion. Dermabraded skin does not heal as well after Accutane therapy. It is important to tell your surgeon that you have been on this drug so that he can make the appropriate decisions about the timing of your dermabrasion.

- Do some planning before choosing this mode of therapy. You will not be presentable for at least a week after the operation. Perhaps, you might consider doing this during a vacation (although I would rather go to Hawaii). It may be three months before people start complimenting you on your new look.

If you decide to proceed, this is what to expect from a typical full-face dermabrasion:

- You will probably undergo the procedure as an outpatient, either in a surgical suite in the doctor's office or in an outpatient surgical center at the hospital. In most instances you will not be given general anesthesia. You could negotiate this with the doctor if you are concerned about the prospect of being awake while someone is planing your face. There is a small but definite risk of serious complications with the use of general anesthesia, even in otherwise healthy people.

- You will be premedicated with agents that will relax you and ease the pain associated with the operation. You may also get a regional anesthetic with what is called a nerve block. The surgeon injects a local anesthetic such as lidocaine into the roots of various facial nerves.

- Once you are anesthetized and relaxed, the operator will begin by spraying a cold material onto the area to be abraded until it firms, much as meat hardens when it is placed in a freezer compartment. This stiffens the skin and makes it easier to run the abrader over it smoothly.

- The skin is then abraded by applying a rapidly revolving electric wheel to the skin and carefully moving this over the face, applying even pressure so that the depth of the abrasion will be uniform.

- After the procedure is completed, your doctor may apply an anesthetic ointment or spray to the treated skin to give you some pain relief. An antibacterial ointment is then applied, followed by an absorbent, nonadherent dressing, which is almost like a mask. At this point, you look something like one of the leading characters in a *Friday the 13th* movie.

- The dressing is left in place for one or two days. When it is removed, you might be better off not looking in the mirror, since your face will be beet red, swollen, and have a crusted surface. After gentle cleansing, a thick coating of an antibacterial ointment is reapplied. This procedure is repeated several times a day so that the skin does not dry out excessively. In spite of your less-than-optimal appearance, there will be relatively little discomfort after the first couple of days. This can be controlled with over-the-counter pain relievers such as acetaminophen.

- After healing is complete, your skin may remain red for weeks or even months, although it usually fades by about six weeks. For a year after the operation, your skin will be thinner than normal, more prone to sunburn, and more sensitive to temperature fluctuations. It is imperative that you avoid the sun whenever possible and use strong sunscreens during the first year.

In competent hands, the rate of major complications with dermabrasion is quite low, but the operation can have problems even when performed by the most skilled surgeons. As noted above, changes in skin pigmentation may occur, particularly in dark-skinned people. This is usually temporary, but it may last indefinitely. Postoperative infections can complicate recovery. This is managed with appropriate anti-infective agents.

The abrasion that occurs on your face is no different qualitatively from that which you might get from skinning your knee after a fall. Just as scars occur after your knee heals, you can have scarring after dermabrasion. This tends to occur around the eyes and along the jawline, but it might happen at any site that is dermabraded.

As with chemical peeling, small cysts (milia) may appear as the face heals. These can be treated by opening them with a small bore needle. Once removed, they rarely will recur.

In patients with oily skin and large pores, dermabrasion may occasionally result in an accentuation of the large pores, particularly in the central part of the face. Repeat dermabrasions may exacerbate the condition. There is no effective therapy for this complication. If you have this type of skin, consider this potential pitfall *before* you undergo the procedure.

Injection of Filling Materials

A popular approach to the treatment of scars and fine lines is soft tissue augmentation. In essence, this is the injection of a substance into the defect to fill in the skin. Several different filling materials are available; each has its advantages and disadvantages.

A perfect substance would be one that would be inexpensive and painless to inject. It would also be inert, so as not to cause a foreign-body or allergic reaction. It would stay in place without shifting its position and would maintain the correction over a long period. Unfortunately, there is no such material. There isn't one that even comes close to that ideal, but there are a few decent alternatives.

All the agents used to fill defects work best at improving shallow scars and fine wrinkles. None of these compounds helps to improve sagging skin, deep-pitted scars, deep wrinkles, furrows, or sunken cheeks.

COLLAGEN IMPLANTATION

The most commonly used material for filling in minor skin defects is bovine collagen, which is available as an injectable gel. Collagen is a complex protein that acts as the scaffolding that gives your skin its structure and strength. This particular variety, marketed under the brand name of Zyderm, is derived from collagen of cowhide. It is changed in certain ways so that it can be injected and so your body won't readily become allergic to it.

This sounds like a great idea; simply place some new collagen in the skin and the structure and integrity will be back to new. Unfortunately, the material does not stay in the tissue indefinitely; rather, it provides a temporary latticework on which your body *may* lay down its own new connective tissue. Sometimes it works, and sometimes it doesn't. In either case the Zyderm disappears after a few months, and usually any correction that has taken place disappears with it. Now, you know the first major drawback of this technology. Most corrections are temporary so you will need repeated touchups if you wish to maintain your new appearance. This can get tedious and expensive, since a single series of injections may cost you hundreds of dollars.

I know the old adage that says that "beauty is in the eyes of the beholder," but I have rarely beheld much improvement in the majority of patients on whom I have used this substance. The patients are often impressed, but after spending the kind of money that they do for these injections, they have a vested interest in good results. Many of my dermatologist colleagues also share my less-than-enthusiastic endorsement of collagen injections.

There are other potential negatives about collagen implantations. About 3% of people are allergic to the material, so an allergy skin test must be performed before it is injected. This is done on the forearm, so if there is a reaction it won't involve a cosmetically important site. If the skin test is negative after three weeks, it is unlikely that there will be a reaction when it is injected into the face. However, there are instances where reactions occur later in therapy, so many doctors will put a second skin test on the forearm even if the first one is negative. This protects against one of these rare adverse events. This all takes time (and money). It might be six or seven weeks after you decide to undergo the procedure before you first get the injections into the affected areas of your face.

Another potential problem with injectable collagen is its possible association with a rare but devastating muscle disease: polymyositis. There have been a few cases of patients developing this disease after getting collagen injections. Whether this is a coincidence or there is a causal link is still being debated.

The treatments themselves are relatively free from problems. The material comes in premeasured syringes containing a local anesthetic as well as the active ingredient. There is usually little discomfort associated with the shots, which are given directly into the scars or wrinkles. An overcorrection is made, so that there is a little puffiness at the sites. This dissipates over the next twenty-four hours. There is often some redness, which also fades by the next day. Occasionally, there is a mild degree of bleeding into the skin, which can leave a bruised area that may take a week to heal.

The big advantage of this form of therapy is that the beneficial effects are seen almost immediately. By the next day, when the redness and swelling have faded, your skin will look better. However, I would suggest that you enjoy it while you can, because the improvement starts to fade away over the ensuing weeks or months. By the end of six months, many people need the first of what could be many visits to the doctor for retreatment.

GELATIN MATRIX IMPLANT

Fibrel is a complex gelatin matrix that provides a lattice that entraps factors that promote new tissue formation. The main theoretical advantage of Fibrel is that even after the material dissipates the new connective tissue network remains in place indefinitely.

This treatment is a little more complicated than collagen injections, in that the gelatin is diluted in some of your own blood plasma. So you have to donate about a half ounce of your blood, a portion of which is reinjected with the gelatin matrix. Your blood has clotting factors that are critical to the success of this product. This is a safe way to get these factors to the spot where they are needed.

If you choose this mode of therapy, your doctor will perform an allergy skin test. However, the incidence of reactions is only about 2%, so it appears that this is a safe treatment.

With all of these positive characteristics, this sounds like a better choice than collagen, but there are major problems with Fibrel. The injections of this material are very painful. Many operators will inject a local anesthetic into the area to be treated before starting the Fibrel injections. Another negative about gelatin matrix implants is that the benefits are modest at best. In one study, only 40% to 45% of scars that were injected with Fibrel were corrected greater than 65%. On the other hand, those areas that do respond tend to keep the correction much better than collagen implants.

As with most things that promise to make you into a new person, this form of therapy is expensive. If you are paying a lot for a treatment that is painful and gives you only marginal results, should you be beating down the door of your doctor demanding it? A dermatologist friend of mine threw a considerable quantity of Fibrel down the toilet after several of his patients complained bitterly about the discomfort and lack of real benefit that they had obtained. Enough said.

INJECTABLE SILICONE

Over the past twenty years, physicians have used silicone to correct skin defects. This has been mostly a cottage industry, since it is technically illegal to use this agent. But an underground market for silicone developed, which led to all kinds of substances being passed off as "medical grade" silicone. It is this impure material that has led to problems with silicone and given this technique a bad reputation. Add to this the huge brouhaha associated with silicone gel breast implants and you are left with a potentially excellent treatment modality that may never legally see the light of day.

When used correctly, this agent comes closest to the ideals I outlined. It is relatively inexpensive, the injections are not particularly painful, the corrections may be permanent, and a variety of skin defects can be treated.

The main problem with silicone is that success is much more dependent on the skill of the physician than its competitors collagen or gelatin matrix. If too much is injected or if it is placed too superficially, the skin can take on a beaded appearance. If inappropriate sites are chosen for treatment, migration of the material may lead to cosmetically unacceptable long-term results. If the compound is injected too superficially in fair-skinned people, the skin may develop a yellowish hue. Another potential uncertainty with silicone is that unsightly reactions may occur years after the injections.

Should you run the risk of using this "underground" drug if the results might really improve your appearance? As a law-abiding citizen, I would advise you to do what the FDA tells you to do. However, if you have a close friend who happens to be a surgically oriented dermatologist and who has wide experience with the use of medical grade injectable silicone, you may want to talk to him about its use.

AUTOLOGOUS FAT TRANSPLANTATION

With the arrival of liposuction, a technique where large quantities of fat are sucked out of subcutaneous spaces, a problem arose about what to do with all of this unwanted adipose (fat-storing) tissue. Some clever surgeon came up with the idea of putting it back into the same person, only in a different location. This was good for the environment (landfills full of fat are quite unappealing), and it did fill in skin defects. However, the early researchers discovered, to their dismay, that the corrections were very transient. The transplanted fat seemed to dissipate.

Over the past decade a great deal of investigative work has addressed the problem of fat transplantation, and some progress has been made. Researchers are still wrestling with the issue of graft survival, however. In one recent study, only 20% of the fat injected into acne scars and 30% of that injected into fine wrinkles survived for up to one year.

Although there are a number of techniques being studied, a similar procedure is followed by most surgeons. Fat is extracted from a donor site somewhere on your body where you don't need it (which means just about anywhere). The material is then injected just below the skin under where the defects are located. With the exception of bruising at the site of the injection, there is little short-term risk with this procedure. Within one day, the skin will look almost normal and the defect will be improved.

This is a technique that may someday be a valuable addition to the cosmetic surgeon's bag of tricks. It would be premature to recommend it now. There is too much uncertainty about the best approach to this treatment. In a few years, this may be a better bet for you.

Hair Transplantation

Slow and steady hair loss throughout life is completely normal in both men and women. Unfortunately, our culture tends to associate baldness with aging, loss of sexuality, and loss of good looks. Current bald-looking hair styles worn by many young athletes have gone against this notion, but most people would probably vote to have too much hair rather than too little.

Modern medicine has come up with an excellent means of restoring a youthful hairline: the hair transplant. Hair is moved from the back of the scalp, a site that usually does not have permanent shedding, onto areas of the scalp where there is no longer any hair. Given sufficient time, new, long hairs grow and cover at least a part of the bald spot.

Hair transplantation is definitely not for everyone who is losing his hair. It does not give perfect results, is time consuming, is expensive, and does not improve your appearance until at least six months after the end of the treatments.

To determine whether you are a candidate for this method of hair restoration, look at yourself in the mirror. If your scalp resembles a cue ball with a narrow surrounding fringe of hair, consider other ways to improve your looks. One needs relatively thick hair in the back of the scalp from which to take the donor hair grafts. If you lack this, there is no place to get the hair to place in the front of your scalp. You are the only possible donor, since foreign tissue taken from another person will be immediately rejected by your body.

In many instances, there is a period of rapid, progressive hair loss which subsides over time. If you are in this phase, you might want to defer hair transplantation until your hairline is better defined. This is particularly true of young men who first lose hair over the temples and then lose it farther back. If you were to transplant the temple areas as they became thinner, your scalp might start to look somewhat weird as the hair behind these new plugs began to fall out, leaving what would look like a row of corn in the front of your scalp. Of course you could undergo several series of transplants as you need them, but the prolonged healing time and general hassle associated with the procedure makes it preferable to undergo only a single series.

If you insist on complete coverage of the bald areas with this procedure, plan to be disappointed. Even in the best of circumstances, hair transplantation will give you a new hairline but not nearly the same thickness that you enjoyed as a young person. In skilled hands, the newly transplanted plugs will be arranged in such a way that you will be able to style your hair to produce maximal coverage. If you plan on seeing how the first session goes before planning future sessions, think again. Nothing looks worse than a half-done hair transplant. The plugs are obvious, and you would probably look better being completely bald.

If you decide to undergo hair transplantation, choose your surgeon carefully. If you can easily tell that someone has undergone this procedure, the surgeon either did not pick his patient well or did not perform the procedure properly. Both plastic surgeons and dermatologists use this technique. There is no particular reason to pick one specialist over the other. Experience is more important than paper credentials in this circumstance.

Although there are several variations on the methods that are used, these are some standard techniques:

- The procedure is usually performed in an outpatient setting. Another person should drive with you to the doctor's office, since you may not feel great at the end of your visit. Your doctor may give you a pre-operative medication to calm you, and this may make you groggy and unable to operate a motor vehicle for several hours afterward.

- The donor area will be clipped or shaven and then cleansed with an antiseptic. You would think that clipping all that beautiful hair before placing it where you need it would be a crazy idea, but all the hairs in the donor plugs fall out after they are transplanted anyway. It will be several months before new hair emerges.

- The donor and recipient sites are then injected with a local anesthetic, such as lidocaine. This hurts, but it is essential. Without local anesthesia, the removal and placement of the hair plugs would be unacceptably painful.

- After the anesthesia has taken hold, the surgeon will remove small plugs (1/10 of an inch) of skin from the bald (recipient) areas of the scalp. This is accomplished with what is called a skin punch, which resembles a round cookie cutter, often attached to a motor-driven apparatus. Next, plugs from the hair-bearing donor area are removed in the same manner and then placed in the holes made in the recipient sites.

- Many surgeons suture the donor areas to control bleeding and facilitate healing. Recipient sites that bleed may also be sutured. A pressure bandage resembling a turban is then applied and left in place for twenty-four hours. The surgeon will probably insist that you return to have him or one of his assistants remove this dressing. At this point the new grafts are not yet anchored in the new sites on the scalp and can be easily dislodged if the dressing is taken off harshly.

- For the first couple of days, there will be some discomfort and swelling. This subsides without anything specific being done to affect it. After about five days, you will be allowed to shampoo your scalp gently. This will dislodge scabs that tend to form around the graft sites. Healing of the recipient areas is usually complete by about three weeks. The donor sites may take some- what longer to heal, particularly if the wounds are not sutured. New hair will begin to emerge from the plugs in twelve to sixteen weeks.

- In most cases, a minimum of four sessions, with fifty to one hun- dred plugs transplanted per session, is necessary to achieve the desired results. These are usually spaced two to eight weeks apart to allow the previous donor sites to heal.

Even in the hands of a skilled and experienced cutaneous sur- geon, unforeseen complications can occur. There may be excess swelling that can affect the forehead and the eyes, leading to "black eyes." These will resolve in about a week. You are not going to look very presentable during this period anyway, so a couple of shiners should not make a major difference in your overall appearance. Although most plugs attach and grow well in their new homes, some- times they can scar and never grow hair. If this happens to only a few plugs, the overall result should still be excellent; however, if a whole row fails to grow, it will affect the ultimate appearance.

There are other surgical procedures that complement hair transplantation; one is scalp reduction. This is particularly useful in patients whose bald area is so extensive that coverage with hair plugs is not practical. When large areas of bald scalp are surgically excised before the transplants are placed, fewer plugs are needed to achieve the desired result.

Another more aggressive means of covering large bald areas is to place a whole flap of hair-bearing skin over a bald zone. A flap of skin is rotated from the back of the scalp to a defect made by cutting away a bald area. This flap is on a pedicle (stalk), which contains the blood supply that nourishes the skin. This is sutured into the site and then establishes itself within a few weeks. This is a much bigger procedure than scalp reduction surgery, and there is more risk of failure. However, the results can be extremely gratifying. You should consider this alternative only if you are willing to do something drastic to change your hairline.

Sclerotherapy for Leg Veins

Spring has finally arrived, and you are dying to work on your tan. (See chapter 4 on the evils of the sun before embarking on this.) After donning a stylish two-piece bathing suit, you note, to your horror, that the barely visible blood vessels on your thighs from last summer now look like ugly reddish blue splotches that even a healthy tan could not cover. This is the occupational hazard of being a middle-aged woman who has given birth and whose mother and sister probably have the same problem. These tortuous, linear red or blue lines are called telangiectasias, or superficial varicosities of the legs.

Before cursing your fate and strangling your children for their part in this mess, consider a procedure that may lighten or even obliterate this troublesome condition: sclerotherapy. The procedure involves the injection of one of a number of irritating materials into the veins, which produces destruction of the vessels. The best results are obtained in the small linear or star-burst-shaped veins on the thighs and legs. Similar veins can sometimes appear on the nose, but these do not respond well to this form of therapy.

In most people, this procedure is devoid of serious complications. However, if you have ever had phlebitis (blood clots) of the legs or a pulmonary embolism (a blood clot that travels to the lungs), you should avoid sclerotherapy. Many doctors prefer to postpone this if you are pregnant, but it can be done in the immediate postpartum period, if you are up to it.

Undergoing sclerotherapy does take some motivation, because there is a fair amount of discomfort associated with the injections and the pain does not come cheaply. Almost no insurance plans will cover the treatment of superficial veins by sclerotherapy.

Several different agents are used, and each has its positive and negative aspects. In the United States, the most common agent used is hypertonic saline, which is a concentrated salt solution. This is effective and is nonallergenic. The main drawbacks are the considerable pain during and just after the injections and extreme localized skin irritation if the material leaks out of the vein that is injected. In addition, some patients experience muscle cramping deep in the area of injection. In Europe, a chemical marketed under the trade name of Aethoxysclerol is widely used. Some physicians in the United States have managed to obtain it, although it is not specifically approved for use by the FDA. The big advantage of this over saline is that the pain associated with the injections is not nearly as severe. There is also less skin irritation if the material leaks out of the vein. It may not be quite as effective, but many people would prefer the slower, less brutal route.

Regardless of which agent is used, the same general procedures are employed. A fine-gauge needle is inserted into the vein, and then a minute amount of sclerosing solution is injected. Many physicians apply a compression dressing over the injected areas for one or two days to enhance the effects of the injected material and minimize leakage out of the injected vessels. Some suggest that elastic stockings be worn, at least overnight, for one to two weeks.

In most cases, several sessions are required to achieve the best results. These are usually given every three to four weeks, because it takes a couple of weeks to see how effective the previous treatment was in obliterating the veins.

Before running to your doctor for this fantastic procedure, note that you might not be completely satisfied with the results. Occasionally, there is persistent brown staining of the skin at the sites of previous injections, which can last up to a year. Scarring can occur if the solution leaks out of the vessels or is injected incorrectly into the tissue around the veins rather than in them. This sounds like an easily avoidable complication, but this is not a simple procedure to master and even experienced clinicians can err in this way.

The success of sclerotherapy is dependent on the expertise of the operator. Many dermatologists and other specialists use this method, and there are no certifying exams or other credentials that separate the expert from the amateur. If it were my legs, I would insist that my prospective leg-vein injector have performed at least one hundred previous procedures before I would even consider letting him inject my veins. When in doubt, personal testimonials from satisfied friends and neighbors are helpful guides in selecting the person to do this work for you.

Laser Surgery

If you are like many of us, you interpret any new technology as one that you cannot live without. There is always a better stereo system, the new computer is always faster and more useful than older models, and high-definition TV has to be better than low-definition TV. So, lasers must be a technology that will revolutionize medicine, simply because they are high tech and on the vanguard. If you believe this, be prepared to part with considerable sums of your hard-earned money because there are some people who would be more than happy to use their new eighty-thousand-dollar laser on your wart or keratosis. The point that I am making here is that not all new technology is necessarily a quantum leap over existing methods of treating disease. With this general warning in mind, there are cosmetic skin problems that can be improved with the laser.

Exactly what is a laser? It is a high-energy beam of a specific wavelength of light that causes tissue damage by producing heat. Depending on the type of light that is emitted from the laser, various kinds of skin diseases can be eradicated. For instance, a birthmark (hemangioma) contains many blood vessels filled with blood that absorbs laser light of a certain wavelength. This light produces intense local heat that destroys the blood vessel without harming the surrounding tissue.

There are a number of common skin problems where laser therapy is the proverbial cannon shooting a flea. If your doctor suggests that any of these conditions be treated with the laser, ask him to also suggest less expensive alternatives or charge you the same regardless of the type of therapy that he uses. Here are a few conditions that can be treated with a laser:

- Skin tags are the small, fleshy growths that occur on the sides of the neck and under the arms. The CO_2 laser can vaporize these tags, but so can an electric needle (hyfrecator). They can also be snipped with sterile scissors or frozen with liquid nitrogen.

- Although warts are not technically a cosmetic problem, many people choose to have them removed because of their unsightly appearance. With the exception of lesions around the nails, the laser should never be the first mode of treatment tried. There are many effective therapies that are inexpensive and relatively atraumatic that you should try before resorting to the laser (see chapter 5).

• Most of us over the age of forty have one or more unattractive brown growths, or keratoses, on our skin surface. As discussed in chapter 5, there are several easy, effective, and inexpensive ways to remove these growths. Don't bother with a laser.

There are a few situations where the laser may be the best possible alternative. One is for the removal of decorative tattoos. The Q-switched ruby laser and the Q-switched Nd:YAG laser both can eradicate tattoos with little or no scarring. These lasers work by sending a beam of light deep into the skin, which pulverizes the tattoo pigment into small particles that are then removed by the body's own blood cells. Several treatments are usually necessary to achieve good results.

If you have concluded that the picture of an eagle on your shoulder does not fit with your image as an investment banker anymore and you wish to have laser therapy, you need to find a practitioner who uses one of the Q-switched varieties of laser. Older CO_2 or argon lasers do not work nearly as well and will guarantee you a scar at the site of your old tattoo. Unfortunately, as of today, there are only a few of the newer-generation lasers available.

Laser therapy is relatively easy to undergo compared with excisional surgery. The discomfort of each pulse of the ruby laser is compared to the snapping of a rubber band or bacon grease splattering on the skin. Some people can tolerate the procedure without any local anesthesia, but many do use some form of numbing medicine locally. Each pulse of the laser treats about one-tenth of an inch of skin. With big tattoos, there may be hundreds of these pulses needed to treat the whole lesion. A session may take over an hour, if the tattoo is large.

There is no reliable way of predicting how many treatments will be necessary to produce a satisfactory result. It may take up to six sessions to clear an amateur tattoo and up to ten treatments to clear a tattoo created by a professional. Those designs with blue-black or green colors tend to respond better, particularly with the ruby laser.

There are few long-term side effects of Q-switched laser therapy for tattoos. Permanent scarring occurs in only about 5% of cases. Occasionally, the skin heals slightly whiter or darker than the surrounding normal skin. There may also be a different texture to the treated skin, which may take on the feel of fine cigarette paper. In many cases, there are some speckles of tattoo pigment remaining, even after many treatments. At some point your doctor will probably advise that the improvement has reached a maximum and that you will have to settle for this small amount of color in the site. At least it won't look like an eagle anymore.

If you cannot locate a physician near you that has access to a Q-switched laser and you cannot live with your tattoo any longer, your next best choice is the CO_2 laser. In most communities, at least one dermatologist has such a machine. This type of laser works by vaporizing tissue, both normal and abnormal. This means you are going to lose the normal skin overlying the tattoo, since the CO_2 laser cannot get to the deeper pigment without destroying the overlying skin.

This therapy requires local anesthesia at the site to be treated. Even the most stoic marine could not possibly stand the pain without it. This proves the dictum that it is a lot less enjoyable to remove a tattoo than to have it placed in your skin, even if you are in a drunken stupor during both sessions.

Unlike the Q-switched laser method, only a single session is usually required to eradicate the pigment. However, because of the risk for significant scarring, your doctor will probably do a small test site and see how it heals over three or four months before attempting to remove the whole thing. I would suggest that you pick the small area that is used for the test site so that you avoid the predicament of one of my patients who had the word BITCH tattooed on his forearm. The test treatment removed the letter "B." Unfortunately, he never returned for his follow-up appointments, so I guess he is going to go through life with a message to the dermatologists of the world: ITCH.

It is not the goal of this form of laser therapy to remove all the pigment in the lesion. In deeper lesions, the tissue destruction would be too severe and the scarring would be unacceptable. Many physicians use an additional method to help tease out the remaining color immediately after the treatment. A paste containing a chemical, urea, is placed on the wound to draw out some of the residual pigment. However, some speckling usually remains as a permanent reminder of your reckless youth. Laser wounds heal quite slowly. It will be three or four months before the scar has healed sufficiently, and it will likely be years before the men in the country club locker room stop ribbing you about your old tattoo.

Index